CUSTOMIZED
CANCER
TREATMENT

OTHER BOOKS BY RALPH W. MOSS, PHD

Integrative Oncology (Ed., with Josef Beuth, MD)
Antioxidants Against Cancer
Herbs Against Cancer
Alternative Medicine Online
Questioning Chemotherapy
The Cancer Industry
Free Radical: Albert Szent-Györgyi
and the Battle Over Vitamin C
Caring (with Annette Swackhamer, RN)
A Real Choice
An Alternative Approach to Allergies
(with Theron G. Randolph, MD)
The Cancer Syndrome

CUSTOMIZED CANCER TREATMENT

Ralph W. Moss, PhD

Equinox Press

Lemont, PA

2010

Published by Equinox Press,
a wholly owned subsidiary
of Cancer Communications, Inc.

Library of Congress Cataloging-in-Publication Data

Moss, Ralph W.
Customized cancer treatment / Ralph W. Moss.
    p. cm.
Includes bibliographical references and index.
ISBN 978-1-881025-01-6 (alk. paper)
1. Antineoplastic agents--Testing. 2. Individual differences. I. Title.
RC271.C5M6685 2010
616.99'4061--dc22
                    2010021935

1 3 5 7 9 8 6 4 2
Printed in the United States of America
on acid-free paper

Disclaimer

The information provided in this book is for general educational purposes only. Neither the author nor the publisher makes warranties, expressed or implied, that this information is complete nor do they warrant the fitness of this information for any particular purpose. This information is not intended as medical advice, and they disclaim any liability resulting from its use. Neither the author nor the publisher advocates any treatment modality. Each reader is strongly urged to consult qualified professional help for medical problems, including board-certified medical oncologists, when appropriate.

Acknowledgements

Many people contributed to the completion of this work. The author would especially like to thank Robert A. Nagourney, MD, and Larry Weisenthal, MD, PhD, for their detailed comments. Any remaining errors are the author's sole responsibility.

CONTENTS

"Current ways of treating people are almost
barbaric compared with what this test can do."
—Robert Fine, MD,
    Director of Medical Oncology,
    The Pancreas Center of Columbia University

"It is far better to study your enemy before the
fight rather than learning as you go."
—*Robert A. Nagourney, MD,*
    Director of Rational Therapeutics,
    Long Beach, California

I. FUNDAMENTALS OF THE TEST

Chemosensitivity and resistance assays (CSRAs) are laboratory procedures in which anticancer agents are brought into direct contact with an individual patient's own cancer cells. By performing CSRA in glassware (*in vitro*) before administering the treatments under consideration, the effectiveness of drugs can be predicted and patients can be saved the time, expense and adverse effects associated with the use of ineffective agents.[1]

For the sake of simplicity, in this book I shall refer to the various forms of CSRAs by a collective name, *the Test*. There are two basic types of such procedures: *chemosensitivity* assays, which judge the ability of drugs to kill cancer cells, mainly through the mechanism of programmed cell death (PCD); and *resistance* assays, which test the ability of drugs to inhibit the growth of cancer cells. For the moment we will consider both tests together, but at a certain point we will differentiate between them.

Model Building

the Test is a form of scientific model building. "Models are of central importance in many scientific contexts," according to the *Stanford Encyclopedia of Philosophy*. "Scientists spend a great deal of time building, testing, comparing and revising models....In short, models are one of the principal instruments of modern science."[2]

When it comes to the life sciences, "certain organisms are studied as stand-ins for others."[3] In the Test, a gram or so of a person's living cancer tissue is studied in the laboratory, where it becomes a stand-in for the actual tumor growing in the patient's body. In this way, the physician can first "treat" cancer outside the body (*ex vivo*), to see how it responds to drugs, before taking the consequential step of introducing toxic substances into a living person.

Bioassays of various kinds are widespread in contemporary medicine, where they are used to measure chemicals in the blood, such as the estrogen (ER) and progesterone receptors (PR) of breast tissue, prostate specific antigen (PSA), as well as tests for fecal blood. There are also tests for the presence of metastases, such as positron emission tomography (PET) or computed tomography (CT), antibiotic sensitivity (the Kirby-Bauer test), etc. Why not, then, an *in vitro* test of cancer cells for their chemosensitivity?

Within living memory, the Test seemed poised for wide-scale adoption. In 1979 the *Journal of the American Medical Association* (*JAMA*) called the Test "almost a reality."[4] Yet in the second decade of the 21st century, the Test faces an uncertain future. In fact, its use has become a matter of disdain to some oncologists. They repeat a familiar mantra: "We tried it, and it didn't work." I was inspired to write this book by one of my readers, who mentioned the possibility of the Test to a loved one's physician:

"This morning during our appointment with my sister's oncologist, we brought this possibility to the attention of her doctor. We were BLASTED all the way up and down as if we were committing a crime of cosmic proportions. The doctor was so mad. You cannot imagine the scene. We are alone trying to treat my sister with something better and every time we try something new we are blasted like this. And I know we are not alone. If you elaborate more, many other people can take advantage of our sad experience, and maybe you can give us more elements to fight back."

It is for patients such as this, as well as for all open-minded individuals, including oncologists, that I have written this book. I wish to show the benefits to be derived from this very good and practical assay, which can be performed *before* the patient undertakes such potentially dangerous treatments as chemotherapy.

The Promise of the Test

Although some oncologists today are dismissive of the Test, this was not always the case. In fact, leading cancer specialists over the years have grasped the huge potential and practical value of this sort of assay:

"The premise of *in vitro* drug response testing is that it can provide knowledge of the relative efficacy of the various agents used in standard therapy before an empiric *in vivo* trial," said John P. Fruehauf, MD, University of California Irvine Cancer Center and Andrew Bosanquet, MD, Bath Cancer Research Unit, 1993.[5]

"Tumor chemosensitivity assays are becoming the method of choice in selecting the best chemotherapeutic agent(s) for cancer patients," wrote the pathologist Sohair Shoman, MD, PhD in his classic book, *Tumor Markers,* 1998.[6]

"The advent of reliable *in vitro* drug response assays has raised the possibility of selecting effective anticancer agents to be used either alone or in combination to treat a patient's individual tumor," wrote Edward Chu, MD, and Vincent J. DeVita, Jr., MD, of the Yale Cancer Center, New Haven, in the latter's textbook, *Cancer: Principles & Practice of Oncology,* 2001.[7]

"My experience with cell death CSRAs [chemosensitivity and resistance assays, ed.] is that they have accuracy in predicting clinical outcomes and defining novel chemotherapeutic synergies. They also have frequent curative value in treating many adult malignancies, which the current medical literature has deemed incurable. I believe that it would be unethical for me not to use such CSRAs in my practice," said William R. Grace, MD, St. Vincent's Hospital, New York, NY, 2004.[8]

"It is an important goal to determine optimal chemotherapy combinations for individual patients to enhance patient response, avoid unnecessary toxicities, and gain insights that may lead to improved treatment strategies," said Patrick Hwu, MD, *et al.*, of the University of Texas M.D. Anderson Cancer Center, Houston, 2006.[9]

"The clinical results of assay-directed therapy are invariably better than would be expected from empirical treatment, but it has proved difficult to get these tests into practice," said Ian A. Cree, MD, Translational Oncology Research Centre, Queen Alexandra Hospital, Portsmouth, UK, 2009.[10]

The National Cancer Institute (NCI) states at its Web site: "A chemosensitivity assay may help in choosing the best drug or drugs for the cancer being treated" (2010).[11]

Despite this open-minded statement, US government-funded research into the Test has ground to a halt, with no immediate prospects for its continuation. I can find no other mention of chemosensitivity testing at NCI's giant Web site (www.cancer.gov). Out of more than 80,000 clinical trials in the US, only four small trials on the topic of chemosensitivity testing are listed at www.clinicaltrials.gov, and all originated from a small private company. Despite nearly $5 billion spent annually on the federal government's War on Cancer,[12] no one at the NCI apparently retains the slightest interest or involvement in evaluating the Test.

Over the past several decades, conventional oncology has gone down a fundamentally different path for selecting drugs. The American Society of Clinical Oncology (ASCO), the main US organization of oncologists, calls this method the "empiric" system. It defines empiricism, in this context, as the "choice of chemotherapy based on the clinical literature describing outcomes achieved when patients receive particular chemotherapy agents."[13] In practical terms, it means the selection of drugs based on the results of randomized controlled trials (RCTs).

For years, the pharmaceutical industry has been researching novel compounds, the Food and Drug Administration (FDA) has been approving some of these as cancer treatments, and oncologists have been utilizing these empirically discovered agents in various combinations in their practices. Thousands of RCTs are conducted every year, many supported by the drug industry, government agencies and private foundations.

Although the results of clinical trials with these agents, by and large, have been disappointing in advanced solid tumors of adults, this may be because patients are poorly chosen for inclusion in such trials. Without knowing in advance who is likely to respond and who is not, many people who have a slim chance of actually benefiting are included in such trials. This leads to disappointing clinical results and brings down the statistical success rate.

Reliance on the results of RCTs to choose a patient's treatment is also deeply flawed, both practically and philosophically. This empiric approach has not resulted in breakthroughs in the treatment of any common form of advanced cancer in adults. *In fact, for most kinds of advanced cancer there has been little progress in the past thirty years.*[14]

I intend to show why the Test offers a better basis for clinical decision-making than empiric treatment.

I realize there are those (such as Scott Ramsey, MD, of the Fred Hutchinson Cancer Center, Seattle) who believe that progress in chemotherapy is slow precisely *because* of a lack of completed RCTs.[15] These authors point to the success achieved in the treatment of pediatric leukemia through the continuous refinement of successive RCTs.

But pediatric leukemia has turned out to be more the exception than the rule among cancer types. It has not proven to be a good model for developing treatments for the far more common solid tumors of adults.*

While RCTs obviously add greatly to the burgeoning store of medical information, these findings provide only a rough guide to what will work for any particular individual. In fact, the more RCTs performed, the greater the

---

* According to the American Cancer Society (www.cancer.org) there were 5,330 cases of acute lymphocytic leukemia (ALL) in the US in 2010, primarily among children and adolescents. This represents about one-third of one percent of the 1,529,560 US cancer cases that year.

glut of *non-personalized information* on potential treatments. I do not think it coincidental that, as RCTs have risen to the fore as the basis of decision-making, progress in treating cancer with chemotherapy (especially for the common cancers of adults) has slowed.

Medical scientists now face a surfeit of scientific data. There is an *information overload*, in which it is difficult for any individual to integrate the many and varied results of clinical trials into an increasingly complex picture. Some think that the solution to this information overload is more and better clinical trials.[16] But in my opinion the empiric method has actually created profound confusion about which drug or drugs, in what combination and schedule, should be given to any individual patient.

Experts in biostatistics are often asked to conduct meta-analyses to sort through this overload of information and to guide the choice of optimum regimens. But even these experts often do not agree, leading to further confusion.

That is because RCTs, by definition, report the statistically average results attained in the treatment of *other people's tumors*. They are not attuned to the peculiar characteristics of a particular individual whose life may nevertheless hang in the balance. Of course, oncologists routinely do modify their prescriptions based on age, tumor size and anatomical location, lymph node involvement, histological grade, and sometimes on patient preference as well. But, except in the last named case, these parameters do not usually affect the *choice* of drugs.

As a general rule, RCTs and meta-analyses are used to choose treatments that are given to hundreds of thousands of cancer patients every year.

Here then are some of the inescapable problems associated with oncology's near-total reliance on the results of RCTs in clinical decision-making:

Individuality of tumors: Tumors vary on an individual basis in their sensitivity to each particular drug, as well as to drug combinations. Even those drugs that are 'well known' for treating particular tumor types (such as platinum-based agents and ovarian cancer) still fail to cause a meaningful response in many individual cases. Consequently, in many clinical trials, the best drugs to emerge from a study do not work for the majority of patients, even "chemotherapy naïve" (i.e., previously untreated) patients. For instance, as I shall show in the case of non-small cell lung cancer, the best empirically discovered drugs only work in about one-third of patients with advanced disease.[17]

To elaborate: "Best" is generally defined as the treatment that causes responses (i.e., shrinkages of measurable tumors by more than 50 percent) or improves the progression-free (PFS) or overall survival (OS) in the greatest number of patients. But in reality even the best regimen chosen empirically will do little or nothing for many patients. For example, in previously untreated breast cancer, patients who receive the "active" drug Adriamycin (doxorubicin), the historical probability of clinical benefit is 50 percent. But this falls to 11 percent if there is an unfavorable finding on the Test and increases to 80 percent with a favorable result in the Test.[18]

Selection bias: Patients enrolled in RCTs may not be representative of patients who are encountered in a typical clinical practice.[19] Because of various inclusion and exclusion criteria, patients in RCTs are generally healthier and more affluent,[20,21] and therefore have a better chance of surviving longer, than do 'real world' patients.[†] "If...the patients in a clinical trial are not representative of the entire patient population because of...selection biases, the generalizability of the results to the entire patient population may be compromised," wrote Karen Antman, MD, past president of the American Society of Clinical Oncology (ASCO), in 1985.

"The prognosis of the general population cannot necessarily be inferred from the selected group in the study."[22,23] Thus RCTs may actually *exaggerate the benefit* of treatment in real life situations.[24]

---

† For example, in Great Britain, people who live in affluent areas live on average *14 years longer* than those who live in poor areas (Shaw, Mary, *et al. The Grim Reaper's Road Map, An Atlas of Mortality in Britain*. Bristol: Policy Press, 2008).

Publication bias: According to some reports, only one-fifth of RCTs are completed and published in peer-reviewed journals.[25] This results in a so-called publication bias, whereby positive results tend to be published in journals, whereas negative ones are either not published or only announced in summary form, through meeting abstracts. This selectivity can also convey an exaggerated impression of benefit.[26]

To summarize then, the near-total reliance on what works for a hypothetical 'average patient' has created a one-size-fits-all, lowest common denominator type of cancer treatment. It would be like saying that since the average male shoe size is 9.5, every man must henceforth wear size 9.5 shoes. RCTs consume an enormous amount of time, money and personnel resources, but they attain results that are not as meaningful to any particular individual as the more expeditious and economical use of the Test.

One hears a lot of talk these days about the need for "personalized," "individualized" or "customized" medicine, but what most oncologists actually practice (at least as far as drug selection goes) is a highly *depersonalized* form of medicine. The process of empiric data acquisition has now pervaded all of cancer treatment.

By contrast, the Test offers an immediate and practical solution to the problem of depersonalization, by customizing treatment based on the unique characteristics of a person's own tumor. It offers not just a better outcome to patients but a path to greater effectiveness and job satisfaction for oncologists.

The benefits of the Test can therefore be summarized as follows:

Patients can be informed in advance which drugs or drug combinations are most likely to kill (i.e., induce programmed cell death in) their own individual cancers and, conversely, which are less likely to do so. Thus, each patient's tumor can be treated in an individualized manner, with their physician employing only those agents that have previously been demonstrated to cause an *in vitro* response.

Ineffective but dangerous drugs can be avoided. "Identification of agents with an extremely low probability of response makes it possible to eliminate the use of such agents and thus their potential for adverse events," wrote Edward Chu, MD and Vincent J. DeVita, Jr., MD of the Yale Cancer Center. "It is intuitively obvious that there should be a therapeutic advantage in the activity of agents to which a tumor is highly responsive *in vitro* as compared with agents that demonstrate significant *in vitro* drug resistance."[27,28]

By eliminating drugs that are unlikely to be effective in a particular case, the patient is subjected to fewer adverse (side) effects.

The Test can provide developmental oncologists (including those employed at pharmaceutical companies) with simple, well-defined laboratory targets by which to judge the likely usefulness of new agents.

Society as a whole can save billions of dollars that are currently wasted on futile, ineffective and highly toxic forms of chemotherapy. In 2006, for instance, cancer chemotherapy sales were $42 billion USD and the market was poised for "staggering growth potential."[29]

A relatively small investment in the Test would yield enormous economic savings later on. By one recent calculation, the Test could reduce the cost of drugs used in conventional chemotherapy from 9.9 to 62.7 percent (depending on the particular kind of cancer).[30]

The Test could shave years off the drug development cycle and new drugs could be made available sooner for customized use. It currently takes, on average, 10 years of research and development (R&D) for a new anticancer drug to reach the market.[31] Society could thus save additional billions of dollars currently spent on unnecessary clinical trials, especially those that at present are performed without a successful outcome, and billions more in the added productivity and longevity of patients.

Whether a drug is "active" or not depends primarily *on the person in question*, and only secondarily on the drug. The actual "best" regimen is the one that is personalized to the needs of the individual patient, and at the present time that can only be reliably discovered through the Test.

II. HISTORY OF THE TEST

It is not my purpose to write a detailed treatise on the historical development of the Test. However, I think many readers would appreciate a brief explanation of its three historical stages of development, for this might help explain the present-day tragic impasse in developing accepted forms of these assays.

In vitro drug response testing gradually emerged from the work of the great 19th century pioneers of microbiology, Louis Pasteur (1822-1895) and Paul Ehrlich (1854-1915). Starting in the 1870s, each evaluated the effects of various agents on the growth of microbial cultures. Ehrlich, who actually coined the word "chemotherapy,"[32] emphasized the need for agents that were selectively toxic. Following this work, Alexander Fleming's (1881-1955) discovery of penicillin in 1929 introduced the modern era of culture and sensitivity testing of antibiotics.

In the 1960s, chemosensitivity tests of antibiotics became widespread in medical practice. The Kirby-Bauer assay and Epsilometer test (Etest) are two such laboratory models used by microbiologists to determine whether or not different antibiotics will kill particular strains of bacteria or fungi.[33,34,35] Subsequent improvements in tissue culture technology paved the way for translating this bacteriological tool to the study of cancer.

Cancer chemotherapy arose in the course of WWII research into the adverse effects of poison gas.[36] In the following decades, the mainstream medical community understood the danger of cancer drug toxicity and the need for chemosensitivity assays to minimize unnecessary toxicity. In 1965, the *Journal of the American Medical Association (JAMA)* editorialized:

"Unfortunately, toxic anticancer drugs inactive against the patient's own tumor may injure the patient by needlessly depressing bone marrow or interfering with wound healing, and by decreasing his 'resistance' to the tumor, thereby enhancing tumor growth... creat[ing] a scientific and ethical dilemma for the physician....A possible solution to the general problem of matching anticancer drugs with the variable chemical requirements of each patient's tumor is 'sensitivity tests for clinical cancer chemotherapy.'"[37,38]

First Generation Tests

Cancer chemotherapy was relatively new when two pioneering doctors, Francis Davis Speer, MD (1909-1987) and Maurice Meyer Black, MD (1918-1996), of New York Medical College, suggested ways of testing drugs *in vitro* to predict their effectiveness in the patient's body. Their first such publication appeared in 1950,[39] followed by several important papers in the mid-1950s.[40,41]

Since I am writing for a non-specialist audience, it is not necessary to go into any of the technical details on how this or any other form of the Test is performed.

Basically, Speer and Black found that a compound called *tetrazolium* would turn red in the presence of malignant tissue, and therefore they invented a tetrazolium dye test. [42,43] Their goal, they said, was to "provide the basis for the clinical usage of tetrazolium as an aid in tumor diagnosis."[44] Overall, their version of the Test proved good at detecting resistance, but weaker in regard to sensitivity.

This was also the first *colorimetric* test for cancer, in that it relied on a change in color of a substance in the presence of malignant tissue.[45] These variations in color, Speer and Black reported, "were distinct and could be defined quite as well as red or colorless."[46] A deep red color was seen in the ducts of all breast cancer patients tested, "while the fibrous and fatty tissue failed to show appreciable color in any case."[47] The color reaction could be made to appear within as little as five minutes, making the test potentially valuable for hospital pathologists performing analyses on frozen sections of cancerous tissue in order to determine the need for surgery.

There was considerable interest in the tetrazolium test in the 1950s and 1960s. Eventually, this test was semi-automated and a machine called a scanning spectrophotometer replaced the visual determination of color. As late as 1988, scientists at NCI and elsewhere were still suggesting that tetrazolium could be used as a means of identifying useful new chemotherapeutic agents or of screening the blood of leukemia patients to detect individual sensitivity to new agents. [48] A form survives as the MTT (i.e., method of transcriptional and translational) assay.[49]

However, despite the initial interest in tetrazolium, it had a number of shortcomings. For instance, there was a "less than optimal sensitivity"[50] due to a variable background color after the reagent was added. There was also a solubility problem. In 1986, European scientists suggested half a dozen ways of overcoming these problems and revitalizing the test,[51,52] but a more fundamental complaint was that this complicated test produced too many false positive results (i.e., finding that drugs would be effective when they were not).

Most American scientists eventually lost interest in tetrazolium, although intrepid Japanese researchers continued to pursue this avenue for several more decades.[53]

One is left with the impression that the tetrazolium test was a very promising beginning, which, although not quite ready for 'prime time,' was an important step in the early development of the Test.

Robert Schrek

There was considerable excitement over some other early tests.[54,55,56] Another pioneer of the Test was Robert Schrek, MD, of Chicago's Veterans Administration (VA) Hospital. According to Larry Weisenthal, MD, PhD, "The exciting things happening right now with regard to drug testing in leukemia and lymphoma could have happened 25 years ago, had anyone paid attention to Dr. Schrek. It would have quickly spilled over also into solid tumors, and we would by now have been way, way ahead."[57]

Schrek tried to correlate the response of lymphocytes in the test tube with the actual clinical responses of patients. But this proved complicated. "Unfortunately," he wrote, this is a difficult problem in view of the many uncontrolled variables in a clinical study and because of the lengthy period required to collect sufficient patients and study their clinical progress."[58] He began the process with a report on the clinical histories of 80 leukemia patients.[59,60,61]

Black, Speer and Schrek were great pioneers of the Test's first generation who anticipated modern thinking on a number of issues.‡ They certainly stimulated the development of reliable versions of the Test, and set the stage for more sophisticated procedures. Their collective

‡ Black was an "energetic and highly committed physician," according to Barron H. Lerner, MD, in the *Breast Cancer Wars* (Oxford: Oxford University Press, 2001, p. 102). He challenged many of the orthodoxies of the 1950s, including use of the Halsted radical mastectomy for most cases of breast cancer. He was also among the first to show that the so-called nuclear grade of a tumor corresponded with the patient's prognosis (ibid.) Schrek, in turn, wrote one of the first articles linking smoking to lung cancer (*Cancer Res.* 1950;10:49-58).

goal was to produce a test that had both a high predictive value for drugs that worked well and the ability to exclude those that did not.[62] Both sorts of information would have been valuable, although the more important (and more elusive) test was the one that could positively identify effective agents.

They knew that a successful assay of that sort would be of incalculable importance to cancer treatment, both for the individual, who often faces agonizing treatment decisions, and for the general field of oncology, including those most concerned with identifying new drugs, the pharmaceutical and biotechnology industries.

In the 1960s and 1970s a great variety of tests emerged, including some in which a patient's cancer cells were implanted into athymic "nude" mice, genetic mutants that have no functioning cell-to-cell immunity and therefore accept human tumor implants. Such experimental mice could then be treated with various chemotherapeutic agents in order to judge their effect on a person's tumors.[63] This was a potentially useful approach, but it was also prohibitively expensive, as each nude mouse cost approximately $50 to $100.[64]

These and other tests had their moments in the sun and were all at one time considered very promising. But their eager introduction was as a rule followed by disillusionment as their limitations emerged. "Although initial enthusiasm existed with each of these assays, it soon

became apparent that their predictive value was not sufficiently specific to warrant broad application," two reviewers wrote in 1985.[65]

Then, in the early 1980s, a new test arrived on the
scene, called the human tumor colony assay (HTCA).[66]
Because of the prestige of its inventors and the journal in
which it was introduced, it quickly rose to prominence. In
fact, it seemed poised to become universally adopted and
to transform the manner in which cancer drugs were
chosen. However, this rapid acceptance was followed by
an almost equally rapid dismissal, an event that still
reverberates through the field of oncology.

Second Generation: Clonogenic Assay

The human tumor colony assay (HTCA)—more commonly
called the clonogenic assay—has been called "the second
significant attempt to develop a reliable *in vitro* drug-
response method."[67]

The clonogenic assay initially generated widespread
enthusiasm. In fact, it still represents what most oncologists are referring to when they speak about (or, more
frequently, against) chemosensitivity testing.

The clonogenic assay was unusual in that it was based
on isolating single human cancer *stem cells*, which many
scientists consider responsible for the ultimate development of tumors.[68] Once a single stem cell was isolated it
could then be grown in a semi-solid medium. Each cell in

the colony was supposedly identical to every other cell, i.e., they were clones. That is why the test was called clonogenic.

It was also a cell proliferation test, which attempted to find agents that stopped cancer cells from *growing* in an uncontrolled manner. Although this appears completely rational, there are basic conceptual flaws to this idea, which I shall discuss shortly.

The inventors of the clonogenic assay were Theodore T. Puck, PhD of the University of Colorado, and his graduate student, Philip I. Marcus, PhD, now of the University of Connecticut. Puck and Marcus initially developed the clonogenic assay in the 1950s as a way of assessing the impact of ionizing radiation on tumor cell growth.[69]

Sydney E. Salmon, MD, of the University of Arizona and Anne W. Hamburger, PhD, of the University of Maryland, later adopted this test to assess the sensitivity of anticancer drugs. Salmon and Hamburger published their procedure, to great acclaim, in the *New England Journal of Medicine* (*NEJM*) in 1978.[70] Not long afterwards, Salmon was appointed director of the Arizona Cancer Center in Tucson.

Early clinical studies using the test as a guide led to "a great deal of enthusiasm and high expectations."[71] In fact, one could say the Salmon and Hamburger publication was a seminal moment in modern oncology, not least because of the implicit endorsement of this prestigious journal. "When the *NEJM* talks," testing pioneer Larry Weisenthal, MD, PhD, later said, "people listen."[72]

Daniel D. Von Hoff, MD, a protege of Salmon, who was then in San Antonio, Texas, became an ardent proponent of the clonogenic assay. A typical paper of those times stated that patients with liver metastases could benefit from chemotherapy if active drugs were selected by means of the clonogenic assay.[73] Von Hoff himself confirmed Salmon's results in a retrospective study.[74]

In one of Von Hoff's studies, responses were achieved by 66 percent of patients who were treated according to the results of clonogenic testing. In these patients there was a 60 percent true positive and 85 percent true negative rate for predicting a response. However, although von Hoff now is among those critics demanding randomized controlled trials (RCTs) from other proponents of the Test, it is noteworthy that he himself never successfully conducted an RCT of the method, when he was a leading clonogenic assay proponent.

Another memorable study was of refractory ovarian cancer, in which 55 percent of patients whose drugs were chosen by the Test responded to their drugs compared to just 18 percent of those who were treated in empiric fashion. The median survival was increased from four to seven months (i.e., a 75 percent increase).[75]

In the early 1980s, there were numerous confirmatory papers on the method[76,77,78,79,80,81] and many private laboratories sprang up to commercialize the clonogenic test. A new day had seemingly dawned for the Test. In 1979, the *Journal of the American Medical Association (JAMA)* enthused:

"The concept of a practical *in vitro* test to predict the sensitivity of various human tumors to anticancer drugs, long an elusive goal of cancer research, may soon become tangible if promising early results from several research centers can be confirmed."[82]

JAMA went on:

"A dependable predictive test of the drug sensitivity of human tumors would play an *immeasurably important role* in the screening and selection of new anticancer agents. Traditionally, the development of such drugs has been a somewhat stumbling process, plagued by uncertainty and expense"[83] (emphasis added).

The basis of the clonogenic assay was to determine which drugs inhibited the *proliferation* of cancer cells. This may seem unexceptional, but, as I have indicated, it was flawed in both concept and design. It was based on a late 19th century idea[84] that cancer in essence is a disease of *unregulated growth*: stop the growth and you thereby stop the cancer. As we shall see, this reflected a faulty understanding of cancer's actual development.

Another limitation was that the clonogenic assay provided data on stem cells, clones of which could be induced to grow in culture. But these elusive stem cells are by most accounts a relatively rare subpopulation of the cancer, and may not be typical or representative of the tumor as a whole or its metastases. In fact, it is not clear what relationship they bear to the rest of the tumor.[85,86]

According to Dr. Robert M. Hoffman of the University of California, San Diego, "Tumors are complex systems consisting of heterogeneous cancer cells as well as normal cells with each exhibiting unique chemosensitivity spectra." He called for "less artifactual, more realistic models [that] can be used to select more tumor-specific drugs which themselves in turn will make *in vitro* chemosensitivity assays more useful for cancer patients." [87]

Thus, the clonogenic test had a major problem with what is now called tumor heterogeneity (discussed below).

The clonogenic assay required three steps: the drugs in question had to be applied to a sample of cells; the cells were then "plated" onto a tissue culture vessel (such as glassware containing circular "wells") and allowed to grow; and the colonies that were produced were fixed, stained and counted.[88] The counting itself was done visually under a microscope, a very laborious process.

No sooner were laboratories established to carry out the clonogenic assay than complaints emerged that

Salmon and Hamburger's test was not all that it was claimed to be. The test proved difficult to set up and execute.[89,90] Some textbooks of the time praised the clonogenic assay as an "*in vitro* system that is a good predictor of human clinical activity...valuable in selecting chemotherapeutic agents for individual tumor types and occasionally specific patients...."[91]

But, in fact, the clonogenic assay was technically feasible in only *20 to 50 percent of selected tumors.*[92] (Evaluable specimens in breast cancer totaled 34 percent, in cervix 20 percent, and in ovarian cancer 52 percent.[93]) In other words, around half the time, the test was a dud. For a cumbersome, labor- and time-consuming test, this was an unacceptably low success rate.

Clinical trial results with the clonogenic assay also proved inconsistent and "reached somewhat divergent conclusions," according to William McGuire, MD, of Emory University School of Medicine, Atlanta in 1994.[94] There were some "extremely promising"[95] prospective studies, but these did not outweigh the practical problems.

There were "overwhelming data" showing that drugs that demonstrated extreme resistance *in vitro* could appropriately be eliminated from the treatment regimen of any given patient.[96] In other words, there was (and is) little debate that ineffective drugs could safely be eliminated from a regimen simply by performing an "extreme drug resistance" assay. (Laboratories, such as Exiqon, still do such testing. See Appendix A.)

But only 41 percent of patients' treatments could actually "be directed by the cloning system results because of inadequate tumor growth and other difficulties." [97] Von Hoff, its most vocal proponent, commented that the results were "encouraging," but "work to improve tumor growth and additional prospective clinical trials of the system are needed before the system can be recommended for routine clinical use."[98]

According to Prof. Robert M. Hoffman, the negative aspects included:

A low frequency of times in which cells could be grown for evaluation;

Clump artifacts in the cell cultures;

A lack of cytotoxic end-points; and

A disruption of normal cell-cell interactions existing in a true tissue environment.[99]

Automated microscopes, flat bed scanners, and sophisticated software were developed to assist in this process. But the problems soon overwhelmed the procedure and conceptual and practical issues led to the abandonment of the clonogenic assay by most of the medical profession.

Dissatisfaction with the clonogenic assay broke into the open at the 13th International Cancer Conference in Seattle in October 1982.[100] Critics complained that the clonogenic assay was plagued by technical problems and appeared to work effectively in only a few types of cancer. Leukemia and lymphoma cells in particular did not grow at all, these critics complained.[101]

In 1985, two researchers summed up their disillusionment but also the hope of the time when they wrote:

"The concept of designing an *in vitro* assay to predict *in vivo* antineoplastic drug activity that would provide the medical oncologist with the necessary data to define beneficial drug regimens is appropriate; however, the optimal assay has been elusive over the last three decades."[102]

Within five years the clonogenic assay was brought low, and with it went the credibility of the concept of chemosensitivity testing as a whole. At the same time, far more accurate tests, based on the conception of what actually constitutes cancer (i.e., programmed cell death) failed to gain traction. Ironically, these superior new tests, which solved the fundamental problems of the Test, were condemned along with the older, less credible clonogenic assay.

"And NEJM Taketh Away"

In 1979, the *Journal of the American Medical Association (JAMA)* had declared sensitivity testing "almost a reality."[103] By the mid 1980s, however, it was a dead duck to mainstream oncology. What happened in the interim? The coup de grace was a "critical appraisal" in the *New Eng-*

land Journal of Medicine in 1985.[104] This *NEJM* article by Peter Selby, Ronald N. Buick and Ian Tannock led to a precipitous loss of confidence in the practicality of the Test and a collapse of the burgeoning *in vitro* assay business.[105]

As indicated, even those forms of the Test that did not depend on analyzing the growth of cancer stem cells went down in this debacle. "Everyone from the NCI on down focused 100 percent of their attention on this single technology," said Weisenthal, in reference to the clonogenic test, "rather than carrying out a comprehensive, head-to-head examination of the whole range of available and proposed technologies.

"When the single technology described in the *NEJM* paper fell short of expectations, everyone became disillusioned and the whole field became discredited, notwithstanding the fact that a whole range of CCDRT [his abbreviation for the Test, ed.] technologies had never been closely examined."[106]

This *New England Journal of Medicine* reversal was one of the most harmful events in the half-century history of the Test. This second publication, coming just a few years after the first enthusiastic report, prompted Weisenthal to wryly comment: "The *NEJM* giveth and the *NEJM* taketh away."[107]

The essence of the 1985 critique in the *NEJM* was this:

The clonogenic assay was unable to support adequate growth in a majority of human tumor types.

It required a large biopsy sample to allow for the inoculation of 500,000 mononuclear cells per plate. This limited both the number of drugs that could be tested and the differing concentrations.

The clonogenic assay used a single concentration of drugs over short exposure time. This raised a number of questions about how well the test mimicked the actual pharmacology of the drugs in question.[108]

Some scientists rushed to rectify these problems in the following few years.[109] In fact, one could say that its failure spurred the development of better tests based on more advanced biological concepts. This included Weisenthal's DiSC assay, which is still in use. But these salutary developments did not seem to matter, as far as the overall field of oncology was concerned.

"The rank-and-file oncologists threw out the whole idea after the [clonogenic] assay proved to be a bust," said Dwight McKee, MD, a medical oncologist in California.[110] Most of his colleagues thereafter equated all cancer-drug response tests with failure.[111] This *NEJM* article led to the current mantra of "We tried the Test and it didn't work."

"The Selby editorial [in NEJM, ed.] killed the field of cell culture testing in cancer," Weisenthal has said, bluntly.[112] "Everyone who had bought and swallowed the

HTCA [i.e., clonogenic assay] sales pitch felt that they had been suckered. Once burned, twice shy."[113]

Weisenthal, who for over 30 years[114] has steadfastly pursued ever more effective forms of the Test, has critiqued the precipitous decline of the clonogenic assay in the mid-1980s, particularly at the National Cancer Institute, where he was a clinical associate from 1977 to 1979:

"Rather than carrying out comparative studies of different types of assay technologies, based on different biological endpoints, the NCI and NCI-funded crowd put all of their eggs in a single basket and did, indeed, shackle the whole concept of culture and sensitivity testing to a single technology. What happened is that the HTCA [i.e., clonogenic assay] technology sank like a stone and dragged the whole concept down to the bottom along with it."[115]

In the mid-1980s, Weisenthal and a colleague reviewed the previous 20 years of clonogenic and non-clonogenic assays. They noted that numerous investigators (such as Sydney Salmon) had stated or implied "with increasing certitude" that clonogenic assays were the most valid (or, perhaps, the *only* valid) approach to predictive chemosensitivity assays.

"Clonogenic assays may not be advantageous compared to other more practical methods of estimating the general chemosensitivity of proliferating cells," they wrote.

By contrast:

"There is a growing body of literature which indicates that early evidence of cell damage in the entire tumor cell population may accurately predict for a multiple-log stem cell kill and meaningful clinical response. Future studies should continue to develop and test assays based on alternative methods for detecting cell kill in the proliferating and total tumor cell populations."[116]

But after the Selby *et al.* review article in the *NEJM*, NCI and its affiliated institutions gradually abandoned the search for improved *in vitro* tests, including those that took into account the sea change represented by programmed cell death. In the US, development of the field was left to a small number of nationally licensed private laboratories. (See Appendix A.)

Some university affiliated chemosensitivity laboratories tried to persevere, but one after another fell by the wayside for lack of financial and moral support. The NCI and its many academic partners went on to other things, mainly (in this area) the vigorous pursuit of randomized controlled trials (RCTs), oftentimes run by large regional oncology groups (SWOG, ECOG, etc.). The RCT became enshrined as the dominant method of discovering and choosing appropriate drugs (both on the individual and the group level), displacing any thought of personalized treatment based on *in vitro* assays.

Weisenthal has stated this about such RCT-based empiric therapies:

"This paradigm seeks to identify the single best treatment to administer to the average patient with a given form of cancer through the use of prospective, randomized trials. I refer to this as the lowest common denominator theory of cancer chemotherapy. Whatever the theoretical virtues of this paradigm, it has been a failure, as established by the last 25 (largely-non-productive) years."[117]

How well these randomized trials work in finding drugs to treat an individual's cancer we shall examine below, concentrating on the case of non-small cell lung cancer.

Third Generation: Programmed Cell Death

Meanwhile, a major paradigm shift was taking place in the scientific understanding of cancer. This discovery in basic science soon created a bright line in the sand between the older forms of the Test and its modern and more effective incarnations.

The new paradigm was based on apoptosis, or programmed cell death (PCD). Its centrality to the field of biological development was recognized in 2002 when the Nobel Prize in Medicine was awarded to three pioneers of the field, Profs. Sydney Brenner of the Salk Institute, John Sulston of the Wellcome Trust and H. Robert

Horvitz of the Massachusetts Institute of Technology (MIT).

Programmed cell death (PCD) has now thoroughly permeated scientific thinking about cancer. In the process, it has also transformed the proper end points for the Test, although that news, odd as it may seem, has failed to penetrate the mainstream oncology community that decides on the acceptability of such tests. In other words, acceptance of apoptosis came too late to rescue a discredited procedure.

The key question is this: Is cancer really a disease of the excessive *proliferation* of abnormal cells? Many people continue to believe this. Even today, decades after the discovery and elucidation of PCD, some dictionaries still define cancer as a "malignant growth or tumor caused by abnormal and uncontrolled cell division."[118]

This is incorrect. Scientists now know that cancer is *not* a disease in which cells grow too abundantly, but as the failure of cells to expire at their appointed time. As Dr. Robert Nagourney has said, "Cancer does not grow too much; it dies too little."[119] Yet the older paradigm of excessive growth persists in many ways. For instance, at its Web site, www.cancer.org, the American Cancer Society (ACS) continues to incorrectly define cancer, in part, as cells that "change and grow out of control."[120]

Almost all basic biologists today acknowledge that cancer is characterized by a failure of PCD. Yet—because one is confronted clinically by an accumulation of the resulting unwanted cells—there remains a strong undercurrent of belief among clinicians that the physical manifestations of cancer must represent *uncontrolled mitosis* (cell division) and that what anticancer agents need to do is stop this wild proliferation of malignant cells.§ Use of this commonsensical (but wrong) definition leads to a dead end in evaluating the Test.

The opening salvo in this paradigm shift was a paper by John Kerr of the University of Queensland, Australia, and two Scottish colleagues, Andrew Wyllie and Alistair Currie of the University of Aberdeen. Writing in the *British Journal of Cancer* in 1972, they described a process they were the first to dub *apoptosis* as a "basic biological phenomenon with wide ranging implications in tissue kinetics."[121]

Kerr initially called the phenomenon "shrinkage necrosis."[122] But the process was more natural and less 'violent' than is implied by the word necrosis, which is a form of *traumatic* cell death resulting from acute cellular injury. So a new word was clearly needed.[123] The word

---

§ By analogy, since the 17th century almost all scientists have agreed that the earth rotates around the sun, and not the other way around. Yet even a contemporary astrophysicist will routinely refer to 'sunrises' and 'sunsets,' implying by his language that the sun revolves around the earth.

apoptosis was derived from an ancient Greek word denoting the natural process by which leaves fall from trees in autumn.** Earlier biologists had repeatedly recognized and described a process very much like apoptosis,†† but without that memorable name.[124,125]

Apoptosis was shown to be an orderly series of biochemical events leading to a variety of morphological changes. Technically speaking, these changes included loss of membrane asymmetry and attachment, cell shrinkage, nuclear fragmentation, chromatin condensation, and chromosomal DNA fragmentation.[126]

The three 1972 discoverers of apoptosis brilliantly anticipated the direction of modern biology when they wrote: "We should now like to speculate that hyperplasia [a category that includes cancer, ed.] might sometimes

------

** Credit for introducing the term goes to a University of Aberdeen Classics professor, James Cormack, PhD, who suggested the ancient Greek word for the dropping off of leaves or petals. Hippocrates used apoptosis in a medical sense to describe "the falling off of the bones," while Galen used it in the sense of a "dropping off of scabs."

†† For instance, in the late 19th century the Edinburgh embryologist John Beard, DSc (1858-1924) described the programmed loss of an entire population of neurons in fish embryos. (Moss RW. The life and times of John Beard, DSc (1858-1924). *Integr Cancer Ther.* 2008;7:229-251.)

result from decreased apoptosis rather than increased mitosis, although we emphasize that we know of no definitive studies to support such a hypothesis."[127]

Definitive studies came later in abundance.

Kerr *et al.*'s initial paper, and subsequent work along these lines, dealt a mortal blow to the idea that cancer was a disease of cellular proliferation. For the last few decades, therefore, cancer has been recognized to be a failure of cellular senescence and death.

The implication of this for the Test was vast, although, as I have said, this fact was not immediately grasped or understood by many. Indeed, like any true paradigm shift, it has taken many years for its implications to percolate down through the oncology community, and it continues to do so.

In the average human adult, between 50 and 70 billion cells die each day due to programmed cell death.[128] In the course of a year this adds up to cells that equal the weight of the individual![129] PCD is also a process with a "strict genetic programme," as H. Robert Horvitz said in his Nobel Prize presentation speech. "The cell death machinery had deep evolutionary roots."[130]

We can trace the progress of the apoptosis concept through the US government's PubMed database. During the entire period 1972 to 1980, there were a total of 35 articles citing the word apoptosis. Now, 50 articles mentioning apoptosis appear in PubMed *every single day*!

The French scientist Pierre Golstein, wrote in the August 28, 1998 issue of *Science:*

"Although there have been scattered reports on the topic of cell death for more than a century, the 20,000 publications on this topic within the past 5 years reflect a shift from historically mild interest to contemporary fascination."[131]

Apoptosis and Chemotherapy

One of the early papers was a 1975 study, with Kerr as senior author, in which certain chemotherapeutic agents were shown to induce apoptosis in mouse tumors. This was an epochal finding, which the authors reported in typically modest fashion: "The significance of the fact that cancer-chemotherapeutic agents induce a type of cell death that is found in normal tissues is at present unknown."[132]

In 1999, John Reed of the Burnham Institute, La Jolla, Calif., extended this observation to cancer treatment as a whole: "Essentially *all traditional anticancer drugs use apoptosis pathways* to exert their cytotoxic actions"[133] (emphasis added).

In retrospect, we can see that this was a landmark finding in oncology. Until Reed's article appeared, most people thought that the nature of the various categories of anticancer drugs (alkylating agents, antimetabolites, microtubule stabilizers, and so forth) sufficiently explained their mechanism of action. But Reed's paper showed that all of these varied agents have a common way of killing cancer cells: in other words, it established "the primacy of survival pathways in human carcinogenesis."[134] Apoptosis and PCD were henceforth seen not as fringe phenomena in oncology—but the way that most anticancer drugs worked. *PCD simultaneously moved to center stage in chemosensitivity testing.*

Since it was turning out that cancer was caused by the *dysregulation* of PCD, advocates of the Test turned their attention to *cytotoxicity*, rather than *growth inhibition*. Focusing on growth inhibition may have identified those anticancer drugs that were unlikely to work, they reasoned, but did not tell which particular drugs were likely to be effective.

While there are many contributing factors to the failure of contemporary oncologists to accept the Test, Robert Nagourney has plausibly argued as follows:

"The medical research community's long fixation upon cell proliferation as the only valid endpoint for laboratory study has led to the development of assay methods which have failed (and continue to fail) to predict clinical outcomes for cancer patients. Tragically, these cumbersome and unreliable methods...have prejudiced oncologists against the entire field of assay-directed therapy and diverted attention away from a lifesaving technology."[135]

The scientific basis of the PCD endpoint in testing comes from a published observation that the most robust cell-death endpoint is *delayed loss of membrane integrity*.[136,137] This endpoint had previously been shown to correlate with both response and survival in human cancers.[138] Detecting this loss of membrane integrity is, quite simply, the principle underlying all the newer PCD-based tests.

MiCK Assay

One scientist who grasped the centrality of apoptosis was the Russian-born pathologist and hematologist, Vladimir D. Kravtsov, MD, PhD. Kravtsov first described his proprietary Microculture Kinetic (MiCK) assay in 1996 (i.e., three years before John Reed's seminal paper). After doing his initial research at Tel Aviv University in Israel,[139] in 1998 Kravtsov moved to Vanderbilt University School of Medicine in Nashville, where he became an Assistant Professor and perfected his MiCK assay.[140]

Kravtsov then licensed his technology for use outside the US to R. Garry Latimer of DiaTech Oncology.[141] Latimer located the company's laboratory on the campus of McGill University in Montreal. In May 2009, DiaTech obtained US distribution rights from the patent holder, Vanderbilt University.[142] Vanderbilt is one of America's top ranked medical research universities and its robust endorsement of this test has been a new high water mark not just for MiCK, but for the Test as a whole.[143] It has potentially begun to revitalize this field and lift the cloud that has hung over it for the past few years.

MiCK is described as "a proprietary laboratory test to help physicians determine specific chemotherapy needs for patients by measuring the response of the patient's own cancer cells to an array of different chemotherapeutic drugs."[144] It is a direct test of apoptosis, and therefore does not rely on any indirect markers of programmed cell death, as some other tests do.

At their Web site (diatech-oncology.com) the company has posted over a dozen published studies on their apoptosis-based test, including some clinical studies. DiaTech is noteworthy for its collaboration with top oncologists, including the surgeon Pat W. Whitworth, MD, of the Nashville Breast Center, Nashville TN and Cary A. Presant, MD of the Wilshire Oncology Medical Group, West Covina, CA.

Beyond Apoptosis

There is some confusion over the related terms "apoptosis" and "programmed cell death." The term "programmed cell death" (PCD) actually predated the word *apoptosis* by eight years.[145] When the idea of apoptosis came to the fore, scientists often spoke of it as synonymous with the older term, PCD. Today it is known that apoptosis, central though it is to biology, is only one of a number of mechanisms that are included in the more general phenomenon of PCD.

"Accumulating evidence suggests that programmed cell death (PCD) is not confined to apoptosis, but that cells use different pathways for active self-destruction," wrote Wilfried Bursch *et al.* of the University of Vienna in 2000.[146] Starting in the 1990s, scientists began to observe various non-apoptotic forms of PCD.

These other forms of PCD include:

Anoikis[147]

Autophagic cell death[148]

Cornification[149]

Excitotoxicity[150]

Oncosis[151]

Paraptosis[152]

Pyroptosis[153]

Wallerian degeneration[154]

The MiCK assay uses apoptosis, but not PCD more generally, as its main endpoint. Nagourney and Weisenthal, and some others, use apoptotic end points, but also include a number of other indicators of PCD (as well as some older tests). The advantages of these are as follows: Programmed cell death end points are more reflective of chemotherapy's actual effects in the human body.

There are peer-reviewed studies that correlate PCD end points with both responses and increased survival.

These tests are 'robust,' i.e., they are both drug- and disease-specific.

The tests are rapid, versatile, and applicable to biologic agents (including even some complementary, or CAM, agents) as well as possibly radiation.

Cytolysis, i.e., the destruction of cancer can be measured in both dividing and non-dividing cell populations.

They accurately distinguish malignant from nonmalignant elements in the tumor.

III. HOW EFFECTIVE IS THE TEST?

The traditional single criterion used to judge laboratory or similar prognostic tests has been the predictive accuracy (sensitivity and specificity) of the test in question. How well does the test predict whether or not an individual will respond to a particular therapy?

One could center an entire volume on the case histories of individuals who have apparently benefited by the Test. While I was writing the present book I received an email from a reader:

"I used Rational Therapeutics' test and my lymph nodes showed that I would be great with Tarceva [erlotinib, ed.] and Avastin [bevacizumab, ed.], which I have been on for almost exactly two months....I just had a scan last week, which showed that the cancer is 75 percent gone! All within 2 months! The tumor had collapsed my right lung, was in both lungs and adjacent nodes; now the lung is almost completely open and the nodes are almost clear, with less nodules in the left lung."

What I find most interesting about this individual's history is that this combination of Avastin and Tarceva had already been subjected to a Phase II clinical trial at Memorial Sloan-Kettering Cancer Center (MSKCC), published in 2008.[155] It was a conspicuous failure, since only one in 38 (2.6 percent) of patients with advanced breast cancer had response. Yet here is a woman with extensive cancer being given a regimen already "proven ineffective" in an RCT and she immediately responds with a 75 percent shrinkage of tumor!

Is this coincidental? That is highly unlikely, given the general "ineffectiveness" of this combination in the RCT. The treatment only made sense because this individual's tumors had already 'told' her doctor that they would respond positively to this treatment.

One could multiply anecdotes of this sort manifold. However, many scientists look down upon case histories of this sort (even when fully documented) as 'anecdotal' and demand a supposedly more rigorous type of proof. One hears a lot about the lack of randomized controlled trials (RCTs) to prove the value of the Test.

There are indeed few RCTs of this method. But there are, by last count, at least *4,263 correlations* that have consistently shown better results using drugs that are active in such tests vs. those that are inactive.[156] There are more than *1,600 published correlations* with cell-death (apoptosis) end points unequivocally proving their clinical utility.[157]

Some of these correlations have also shown increased survival in such patients. Ordinarily, this would be sufficient to establish the merit of a test and justify Medicare, Blue Cross/Blue Shield and other insurers to pay for it. (The lack of reimbursement is the key practical impediment to the dissemination of the Test.)

For critics of the Test, however, this abundance of correlative data is not enough. The doctors who conducted the ASCO review of the Test in 2004 deliberately and explicitly *excluded* all papers showing a correlation between the Test's predictions and patient outcomes!

In the words of these ASCO reviewers:

"We excluded reports that only reported correlations between assay results and clinical outcomes"[158] (where "outcomes" refer to both responses to treatment and patient survival). I shall say more about this faulty ASCO evaluation below.

Oncologists' insistence on the necessity of randomized controlled trials demonstrating increased progression-free (PFS) or overall survival (OS), although reasonable-sounding, turns out to be a rather strange demand. As Weisenthal points out:

"There has never been a laboratory or radiographic test in the history of medicine that has been shown to confer a treatment benefit in prospective trials in which patients were randomized to treatment with and without benefit of the tests."[159]

Therefore the refusal to recognize or financially compensate for the Test until successful survival-oriented RCTs are completed constitutes an "illogical, unreasonable, and unprecedented barrier to the more rational management of such a serious disease as cancer."[160]

I need to re-emphasize Weisenthal's crucial point. To his knowledge (and he has been an active participant in the development of the Test for more than 30 years[161]) there has never been a randomized trial "proving" the therapeutic benefit of *any* laboratory test including, of course, any previous drug resistance assay.

This was true of early tests (such as the now standard test for the estrogen receptor, ER, in breast cancer or the prostate specific antigen, PSA, in prostate cancer) as well as for newer molecular or genomic assays, such as the increasingly popular Oncotype DX™ test for breast cancer. In fact, in marked contrast to the Test, the Oncotype DX™ test, despite the lack of RCTs, has been approved both by ASCO and the National Comprehensive Cancer Network® (NCCN), an alliance of 21 of the world's largest cancer centers.‡‡

All that proponents of these other *in vitro* tests had to do was to demonstrate their *accuracy*. They did not need to prove their *effectiveness,* in the sense of conducting rigorous trials showing that use of their procedure increased patients' survival.

The Test is essentially a laboratory *tool*. Like any tool, it should be judged by its craftsmanship. It is then put in

‡‡ In 2010, the NCCN issued a "category 3" recommendation for CSRA in ovarian cancer. This acknowledged that some of its member centers were using the test.

the hands of individual practitioners, who vary in terms of their skill and competence. But, unless it is defective, the tool itself cannot be held responsible for the results achieved, any more than a well-crafted hammer can be faulted if an unskilled carpenter builds a house that falls down.

There are three main ways that one can judge the validity of *in vitro* assays such as the Test:

Retrospective comparisons of test results with patients' *responses* to therapy.§§

Retrospective comparisons of test results with patients' length of *survival*.

Prospective randomized controlled clinical trials (RCTs) comparing standard therapy with chemotherapy chosen by *in vitro* assay results.

The invariable argument used to deny the validity of the Test is that only the first two types of data, but not the third type, support its use. The first two types supposedly do not have the same 'rigor' as large, multi-center phase III randomized trials.

---

§§ According to the standard WHO/IUCC criteria, a partial response in oncology is generally defined as a decrease of 50 percent or more in the entire tumor burden. Some have suggested that a 30 percent shrinkage is sufficient to qualify as a partial response (*Jpn J Clin Oncol*. 2004;34:740-746).

But in a comprehensive 1999 review, Fruehauf and Bosanquet (writing in an update of the DeVita textbook) agreed with Weisenthal's argument, as follows:

"The first two comparisons are the *normal methods* by which laboratory tests are assessed for accuracy. Many have called for prospective clinical trials, even though other laboratory tests (the results of which also guide clinical decision making) seldom are assessed in this way"[162] (emphasis added).

Weisenthal admits that the Test "has never been shown, in prospective randomized trials, that there is a clear advantage to chemotherapy selected with the benefit of knowledge of the CCDRT [his abbreviation for the Test, ed.] results compared to 'physician's choice' chemotherapy selected without knowledge of the CCDRT results."[163],*** As Chu and DeVita point out, however, conducting an adequately powered RCT of chemosensitivity tests with survival as an endpoint would be fraught with all sorts of unique difficulties. For instance, "the

***

*** This was written in 2003, four years before the small RCT by Cree *et al.* from Plymouth, England (discussed below). The Plymouth RCT demonstrated an improvement of both response and progression-free survival in the arm that was guided by the Test, although it was apparently underpowered to detect overall survival advantages in this advanced a patient population. This is frequently a problem with clinical trials that are too small to establish their own basic premises.

efficient procurement of tumor tissue remains a serious problem."[164]

What they are apparently alluding to is that even in the normal course of events patients who request the Test are often frustrated by uncooperative surgeons and physicians. Many doctors refuse to facilitate a test that they do not believe in. Others, after initially agreeing to cooperate, fail (a) to procure an adequate amount of living tissue, (b) to preserve this tissue in a viable condition, or (c) to expedite its delivery to the testing laboratory. In any one of these ways, an uncooperative doctor anywhere along the chain of delivery can undermine the successful completion of the Test.

The demand for an RCT to prove the validity of chemosensitivity testing is therefore:

Abnormal under the circumstances, since it has not been required of other approved tests;

Unnecessary, since retrospective data correlating patient responses and survival with test results provides sufficiently accurate information for Medicare, Blue Cross/Blue Shield and other insurers to approve such a test; and

Impractical, since experience shows that there are insufficient resources or enthusiasm in the oncology community to conduct such a trial.

In fact, in the 1980s, Weisenthal twice tried to organize rigorous trials in the regional oncology groups. He failed both times, not because of any deficiency in the assays themselves, but because of poor accrual of patients.[165]

the Test is therefore being asked to perform to a standard that is more stringent than necessary, in fact more stringent than any other laboratory test in the history of medicine. It is a classic instance of a double standard.

It is only when these tests are put on a par with all other laboratory tests – that is based on their "accuracy" and not their "efficacy"—that their use is likely to become more broadly available. The mantra-like demand for a randomized trial for the Test is often disingenuous as well. That is because many of the individuals or groups that raise this issue (some of whom are exceptionally well-funded with taxpayers' dollars) are not willing to pay for such a trial. In colloquial terms, *they do not put their money where their mouth is.*

Classification of Drugs

Larry Weisenthal has summarized the results of 50 completed non-randomized clinical trials, as well as 500 or so published clinical correlations. On this basis, he has classified all anticancer drugs into four categories:

Category 1: Drugs that have virtually no chance of working for a particular individual;

Category 2: Drugs that have a lower than expected chance of working;

Category 3: Drugs that have an average chance of working; and

Category 4: Drugs that have a higher than expected chance of working.

By analyzing a large array of published studies, conducted over three decades, he reached the following conclusions.

All other factors being equal, he says, there is a:

- 20:1 advantage in choosing category 4 drugs over category 1 drugs;
- 10:1 advantage in choosing category 3 drugs over category 1 drugs;
- 2:1 advantage in choosing category 2 drugs over category 1 drugs;
- 2:1 advantage in choosing category 4 drugs over category 3 drugs;
- 7:1 advantage in choosing category 4 drugs over category 2 drugs; and a
- 3 or 4:1 advantage in choosing category 3 drugs over category 2 drugs.[166]

The Use of Correlations

What then is the scientific basis for claiming that the Test is an effective method for choosing drugs?[167] As stated previously, John P. Fruehauf, MD, and Andrew G. Bosanquet, MD, writing in an update to the DeVita textbook, found a total of 4,263 clinical correlations of the Test with outcomes in the medical literature.[168]

How did these patients perform in their response to chemotherapy when their treatment was guided by the Test's results? The authors found that, on average, there was an *overall sensitivity of 85 percent* and an *overall specificity of 80 percent.*

These are the standard terms by which clinical tests are judged. But since they may not be familiar to the general reader, I need to define them in greater detail.

First one must understand that there are four possible responses to the Test. These are (1) true positives, (2) false positives, (3) true negatives and (4) false negatives (See Table 1).

Table 1

Possible Responses to the Test

	Disease Present	Disease Absent
Test Positive	True Positive (TP)	False Positive (FP)
Test Negative	False Negative (FN)	True Negative (TN)

Source: Martens, 1995

Sensitivity refers to the ability of a test to *rule in* what it is being sought (in this case, a particular drug for a particular patient). When we say that a test has an overall sensitivity of 85 percent, we are saying that 85 percent of patients who are actually sensitive to drug A test positive for that drug.

The appropriate formula for finding this number is Sensitivity = TP / TP + FN. In statistics, "TP" is the number of true positive results. It is then divided by a combination of true positives and false negatives to reach the sensitivity rate.

Sensitivity (which is also called the recall rate in other fields) measures the proportion of actual positive results that are correctly identified as such. For example, it might be used to specify the percentage of sick people who are correctly identified as having a particular condition.

Specificity by contrast measures the proportion of negative results that are correctly identified. This might be the percentage of healthy people who are identified as not having the condition.

Put another way, *specificity* is defined as the ability of a test to *rule out* what is not there to be found. It refers to the proportion of patients who have a true negative (TN) result. The formula in this case is Specificity = TN / TN + FP (or true negatives over the combination of true negatives and false positives). For any given test, then, the numbers for sensitivity and specificity define the performance characteristics of the test, i.e., how well the test does its job.

RALPH W. MOSS / 65

In theoretical terms, the world's best predictive test would have a sensitivity rate of 100 percent if, say, predicted all people from a sick group as being sick and 100 percent specificity, if it did not predict anyone from the healthy group as being sick.

"Sensitivity, specificity, and positive and negative predictive accuracies are used to define any test's utility," said Robert Nagourney "and according to established standards."[169]

The question then is, how well the Test actually performs in regard to sensitivity and specificity. How does it compare in this regard to other standard tests? As many independently verified sources make clear, the Test's accuracy rate, while not perfect, is very similar to (or better than) the rest of the standard and accepted tests in use today.

Here for example are two charts, which I have somewhat modified from data and graphics provided in a 1999 textbook. They show that the Test actually has a somewhat *higher true positive* rating than such familiar tests as for estrogen receptors, bacteria sensitivity, or fecal blood (Chart 1).[170]

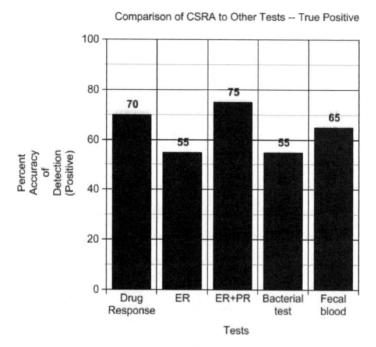

Chart 1

the Test's *true negative* rate is also similar to that of all of these standard tests (Chart 2).

Chart 2

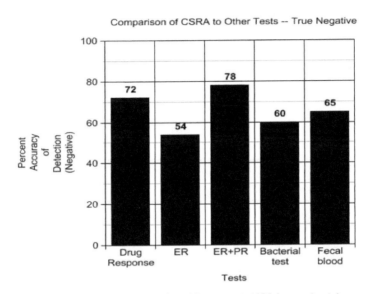

Comparison of CSRA to Other Tests -- True Negative

Fruehauf and Bosquanet, 1999 (approximate)

By these standards, many forms of the Test, particularly those using programmed cell-death (PCD) end points, perform *better* than most conventional tests. Yet, as I have shown, the Test is *not* being evaluated by the same standards as ER, PSA, or these other tests, but is being held to an impossibly higher standard.

Comparison to ER Test

I now want to discuss the question of estrogen receptor (ER) testing in greater depth, since it is such a well-known and well-accepted test. I will then compare the oncologists' acceptance (indeed reliance on) ER testing with the near-total rejection of the Test.

It was noted in the 1960s that some women with breast cancer underwent "striking regression after surgical removal of glands" that were responsible for the production of female hormones; many did not respond, however.[171] Receptors that bound to the female hormone estrogen were soon discovered in the reproductive tissue of experimental animals. It was then found that these receptors were also more copious on the breast cancer cells of patients who responded positively to hormonal ablation (i.e., removal or destruction) than were the tissues of non-responders.

In the 1970s scientists therefore began to measure estrogen receptors on breast cancer tissue in the laboratory and used these scores to predict an individual patient's responsiveness to such anti-hormonal therapy.[172] A standardized test was self-evidently beneficial in identifying likely responders and sparing the many non-responders the rigor of anti-hormonal treatment (which then consisted of adrenectomy, hypophysectomy or, in premenopausal women, ovarian ablation).

The ER test was originally a complicated biochemical test called the "radioligand binding" (RLB) assay.[173,174] This was validated in the late 1970s and early 1980s by means of retrospective correlations between the clinical outcome in patients who were treated with anti-hormonal therapy. There were no randomized controlled trials (although the RCT was, by that time, *de rigeur* for new drugs).

A typical report of the time, from the University of Chicago, stated: "On the basis of 134 treated patients, nearly two-thirds of the receptor-rich group can expect objective benefit from endocrine therapy, whereas few if any of the receptor-poor patients will respond."[175]

Most oncologists agreed that "the determination of hormone receptors in primary or metastatic breast tumors is at present the most reliable test in selecting breast cancer patients for endocrine therapy."[176]

But remember that patients with a tumor that scores "positive" in an RLB assay had about a 60 percent chance of responding to hormonal therapy. A tumor that was negative on RLB still had a 10 percent chance of responding to anti-hormonal therapy.

The test was approved because it addressed "a basic clinical problem: how to determine which cancers are hormone dependent without an actual treatment trial."[177] It simply fulfilled a felt need for choosing good candidates for ablative surgery (and later for anti-hormonal drug therapy).

Particularly noteworthy is the fact that even the simpler tests for ER receptors was never proven effective *at extending survival* through phase III RCTs before being put into general use. Luckily for the hundreds of thousands of women who have benefited from this test, such an onerous demand was never raised in the case of ER+ detection tests. These tests fulfilled the demand made of all laboratory tests throughout history: it was accurate and reasonably sensitive at finding good candidates for a particular therapy.

Once the ER test received wide-scale acceptance and approval, scientists naturally worked on improving it. The original RLB assay could only be performed at highly specialized laboratories and was eventually replaced by a so-called immunohistochemical (IHC) test.[178] But this too was not subjected to randomized controlled trials (RCTs) before being implemented nor was it ever independently validated as a predictor of response to hormonal therapy. It was merely compared to the previous test, the RLB, which was more cumbersome and therefore less desirable.

Although the new ER test was not rigorously evaluated, nevertheless, it was "quickly moved out into hundreds (possibly thousands) of community hospital pathology laboratories," as Weisenthal has said. Despite the lack of rigorous studies (much less studies demonstrating increased survival by using the test) "hundreds of thousands of cancer patients have had life and death treatment decisions based on these tests."[179]

Finally, many years later, there was a published study on the ability of the IHC test for estrogen receptors to predict a patient's actual clinical response to hormonal therapy.[180] In this study, from Nagoya City University Graduate School of Medical Sciences, a total of 75 patients with metastatic breast cancer were studied. They all received first-line treatment with endocrine therapy (the drug tamoxifen, etc.)

It turns out that the ER test was not as accurate as previously thought. It was certainly not as accurate as the current generation of chemosensitivity testing using PCD end points. The authors of the Nagoya study reported that there were 15 patients with both estrogen (ER) and progesterone (PR) negative tumors, and 3 patients (20.0 percent) responded to tamoxifen therapy.[181] Conversely, "The ratio of responders with both ER- and PgR-positive tumors was 56.8 percent."

In other words, *only slightly over half* of those with a positive ER score actually responded to anti-hormonal treatment. And this was from a laboratory that, as part of a long established academic center, had above-average experience in utilizing this "standard" test in the treatment of breast cancer. One can only imagine what the accuracy of this test is in the various small community hospitals around the world where it is also commonly employed.

Please do not misunderstand me. I am not raising these points in order to denigrate the ER receptor test. It is perfectly adequate, and has been highly beneficial to countless patients. Nevertheless, it has its limitations, as all tests must. What is striking is the entirely different manner in which ER receptor assays have been handled 30 or 40 years ago compared to the demands currently being made of the Test proponents.

The sensitivity and specificity of the third generation of the Test are much higher than any standard test for ER receptors. Nevertheless, the Test has been rejected out of hand by the oncology community, which has embraced the far less accurate ER assay. There is thus a double standard at work, which is not only unfair but is crippling prospects of the Test.

Comparison to PSA Test

I cannot let this topic go without also making a further comparison to the familiar prostate-specific antigen test (PSA) for prostate cancer. The traditional upper normal limit for the PSA test is 4.0 nanograms per milliliter (ng/mL) of blood. When this level of PSA is chosen as the upper boundary of normal, only 20 percent of all men who actually have prostate cancer will be recommended to have a follow-up biopsy.[†††] So, the historical level of 4.0 ng/mL fails in its primary goal of a cancer screening: find-

---

[†††] In the case of the more aggressive high-grade (Gleason grade 7 and higher) disease category, the results are somewhat better. A level of 4.1 would actually find *40 percent* of those men with more aggressive cancers.

ing a high percentage of those men harboring occult forms of the disease.[182]

According to a much-cited article in the *New England Journal of Medicine,* biopsy-detected prostate cancer "is not rare among men with PSA levels of 4.0 nanogram per milliliter or less—levels generally thought to be in the normal range."[183]

Again, my point is not to criticize the PSA test, which is a very useful tool for urologic oncologists. But the PSA test (like the ER and many other tests) were evaluated and accepted on the basis of the accuracy of their *correlations* between test scores and patient outcomes (either responses or survival). One can endlessly debate the utility of these tests. But as the reader can see, the sensitivity and specificity of both of these assays falls short of what has been repeatedly shown for the Test, especially in its modern incarnations.

Yet, as I have shown, *correlations* in general were explicitly *excluded* from the fateful ASCO review of 2004. The only valid appraisal, the world was told, was based on how well the Test performed in extending survival, as demonstrated through non-existent randomized controlled trial (RCT).

This was the type of trial that Daniel Von Hoff, the member of the ASCO panel with the greatest experience with the Test, had himself failed to ever conduct for his own method of choice, the clonogenic assay, during the decades that he championed that test.

Ironically, in 1990 Von Hoff himself was in the fore-front of those pointing out the impracticality of such a clinical trial:

"An ongoing randomized trial in which investigators are attempting to corroborate these results in patients with previously untreated small cell lung cancer has been so slow to accrue patients that it is unlikely these trials and others will ever be completed."[184]

Indeed! Yet 14 years later Von Hoff himself was among those demanding the same rigorous trials from his erstwhile collaborators.

That is why I say that the ASCO reviewers' call for RCTs was and is disingenuous, since they know full well that the proponents of third generation tests have no ability to perform these tests and they themselves have no intention of performing them either. In fact, the ASCO report has spelled the death knell for the acceptance of the Test for years. As Weisenthal said, this demand for large-scale RCTs proving "validity" (as opposed to accuracy) "has been disastrous with regard to the goal of personalized medicine in cancer treatment."[185]

Microspheroids

There are a number of variables that affect the helpfulness of drugs. These include the rate of excretion of these drugs by the kidneys and liver, protein binding, and a myriad of other biological factors. Another issue is the fact that some anticancer drugs are actually pro-drugs, which need to be first activated in the liver before becoming biologically active. Thus, *in vitro* testing laboratories must administer the *active* forms of these agents, not the pro-drug form that is given to patients.

In the past, researchers of the Test usually tested cancer cells in isolation, in single cell suspensions. Somehow it was thought that the individual cell (particularly if it were a stem cell) represented a 'purer' form of the cancer. This turned out to be a mistake, since cancer cells isolated in a test tube simply do not behave in the same way they do when growing in the human body.

In the body these cells interact with—and are supported by—myriad other living cells, both malignant and normal. That is the reason that some laboratories using the Test now study cancer cells in small clusters, or microspheroids. Analysis of these microspheroids provides a "snapshot" of cancer's behavior within the human body and provides a more accurate representation of how cancer cells are likely to respond to treatment in the clinic.[186] It is crucial that there is no manipulation of the isolated cancer cells to make them grow, an important point of distinction with earlier tests.

Boris Rotman, PhD, a biologist at Brown University, then affiliated with the Analytical Biosystems Corp., first enunciated this crucial microspheroid concept in the mid-1980s.[187] Rotman developed a Fluorescent Cytoprint Assay,[188,189] which relied on what he called "micro-organs." He cited preserving cell-to-cell interactions present in the original tumor" as an advantage of his test.[190]

In 1992, Larry Weisenthal adopted this concept and began analyzing microspheroids in *all* of the chemosensitivity testing he performed in his laboratory. He carried this concept further, applying the term "microclusters" (which had previously existed in a different context[191]) to the end product of the method of tumor dissociation that he had developed. This same technique is currently employed at Nagourney's Rational Therapeutics as well.

Long experience has shown that cancer is, in essence, a "social animal." Real-life cancers grow as a complex organism that includes both malignant and non-malignant components. It may include fibrous tissue, mesothelial cells, fibroblasts, endothelial cells, etc. In order to exhibit its most characteristic behavior patterns, a cancer cell needs to be surrounded by a colony of other cells, both normal and malignant.

Here is how Robert Nagourney, in rather technical terms, described this formation in a 2008 presentation to the American Association for Cancer Research (AACR):

"Human tumors represent micro-ecosystems composed of transformed cells, stroma, fibroblasts, vascular elements, extra-cellular protein matrices and inflammatory elements. The behavior of human cancers and their response to therapy reflect the complex interplay between humoral, vascular, adhesion and cytokine-mediated events acting in concert."[192]

His basic point is that tumors are clearly very complex organisms. Ignoring this complexity, most studies of human cancer in culture have focused upon individual tumor cells that have been removed from their complex microenvironment. Cells are routinely broken up by mechanical and enzymatic means, which alters their subsequent behavior. Some of the previous methods of the Test limited their analysis only to isolated tumor cells, and failed to incorporate the "crucial contribution of non-tumorous elements"[193] to the cancer phenomenon.

"These assays have proven incapable of providing clinically relevant predictive information," said Nagourney.[194] He points out that when allowed to grow *in vitro,* living cancer cells develop into these tiny micro-spheroid clusters that form a complex biosystem, in which each malignant cell reacts upon its fellow colonists in subtle but important ways. Each of these microspheres contains "all the complex elements of tumor bio-systems that are found in the human body and which can impact clinical response."[195]

In my opinion, this observation has not received the attention it deserves. But this orientation is similar to that of Mina Bissell, PhD, Distinguished Scientist at the

Lawrence Berkeley National Laboratory/University of California. Bissell has spent her career researching the role of the extra-cellular matrix (ECM) in the growth of breast cancer. According to her Web site, her work has "strengthened the *importance of context* in the development of cancer" (emphasis added). After decades of rejection, Mina Bissell was awarded the American Cancer Society's Medal of Honor in 2008.

Bissell has made what amounts to a powerful critique of genetic determinism regarding cancer. As she told a reporter, if cancer were the inevitable outcome in any cell carrying the "breast cancer gene," why then don't people with that gene develop cancer in *every* part of their bodies, not just the breast? "And why is it that breast cancer develops in adulthood if the gene mutation has been there all along?" she asked. If inheriting a single DNA mutation were enough to cause cancer, one's entire body should be cancerous, since the complete genome is present in each somatic cell. "You would be a lump!" she exclaims— "a gigantic tumor."[196] Clearly something else is involved, and that 'something' is the cellular microenvironment and the extra-cellular matrix in which the individual cancer cell grows and thrives.

Analyzing isolated individual cancer cells is no more meaningful than an anthropologist analyzing an individual subject removed from the context of his or her society. This is a *crucial distinction* between modern-day chemosensitivity testing and the older technology. It is also a crucial difference between the newer molecular analyses, which some people think has supplanted the need for analyzing actual colonies of tumor cells. But genomic analysis has yet to confront, much less solve, the question of establishing an *in vitro* model that truly reflects the behavior of cancer cells in the body.

In the past, the effectiveness of the Test was hampered by a lack of knowledge of how cancer actually behaves in the living individual. This is gradually being overcome as the science of oncology progresses in its understanding of the tumor's relationship to its microenvironment.

Heterogeneity of Tumors

One issue that is often raised in regard to the alleged limitations of the Test is the so-called heterogeneity of tumors. This means that primary cancers and their metastases, in real life clinical situations, are not made up of exactly identical cells (or clones) and so therefore may not consistently respond to the same agents.

This sort of inconsistent response is sometimes seen in clinical practice. For instance, a tumor in one location may respond to treatment, while other tumors (or metastatic colonies) in the same person do not. There is one report on the clonogenic assay stating there is a 32 percent discordance rate between the responses at different tumor sites in the same patient.[197]

I have been unable to find confirmation of this statistic elsewhere in the scientific literature. Oncologists who treat cancer patients tell me that they sometimes do see metastases responding to treatment while primary tumors remain stable, or vice versa, but that it is rare to find one tumor growing while another one is shrinking.

According to Nagourney, tumor heterogeneity is a real issue. This is because cancers are complex entities encompassing what are called 'clonal variants.' These may have different degrees of sensitivity to drugs. The above reference to heterogeneity in the clonogenic assay results is "not terribly interesting," he adds, because we know, beyond a shadow of a doubt, that tumors have differing proliferative indices within the same tumor population.

Thus, when you force tumors to grow, they will certainly manifest different "growth inhibition" profiles. This means that the most proliferative cells would also be the most sensitive to the anti-proliferative effects of most drugs. While this becomes much less of an issue in programmed cell death (PCD) based assays, in which tumors are not being propagated, "it is still a theoretical and possibly clinically relevant point."[198]

"This question is critical," wrote Massimo Cristofanilli, MD and John Mendelsohn, MD of the University of Texas M.D. Anderson Cancer Center, Houston (where Dr. Mendelsohn is President), "because it is widely accepted that cancer cells that have spread to different metastatic sites express different genes and may harbor different genetic abnormalities."[199]

For example, in 2004 Meng *et al.* of the University of Texas found that patients' circulating tumor cells (CTCs) could exhibit over-expression of the HER-2 gene, even though their primary tumors did not do so. Nine of 24 breast cancer patients, or 37.5 percent, whose primary tumors were HER-2-negative acquired HER-2 gene amplification in their CTCs during the progression of their disease. Four of these nine patients, who ordinarily would not have been considered candidates for the drug Herceptin (trastuzumab), which targets HER-2 over-expression, were then treated with Herceptin-containing therapy. One of these then had a complete response and two had a partial response.[200]

Thus, cancers may acquire new characteristics as they progress, circulate in the bloodstream or proceed to form distant metastases. This is a sign of heterogeneity within an individual's cancer.

Nagourney points out that tumor heterogeneity is a fact with which *any and all* tests and drug protocols must contend. It is not limited to regimens designated by the Test. For instance, in April 2010, Gina Kolata of the *New York Times* detailed the nightmarish situation of breast cancer patients, parts of whose tumors over-express Her/2 protein, while other parts do not. Are such patients Her/2 neu positive or negative? The tests are often ambiguous.

As Kolata says, "[W]hile most patients do not yet know it, those tests can be surprisingly unreliable" and "the problem continues to grow."[201]

But this problem of tumor heterogeneity, Nagourney says, cannot possible be worse with the Test than it is with empiric therapy, which to chemosensitivity testing advocates represents mere guesswork. Nagourney agrees with his colleague, Larry Weisenthal, that "most patients either respond or do not respond to drugs." So, practically, heterogeneity remains a rather small clinical problem. These so-called "mixed responses," while theoretically possible, are relatively rare.[202]

There is a possible way around the problem. When oncologists, guided by the Test, select drugs and deliver therapy they tend to eliminate the predominant clones in the tumors. Once that is done, and the tumor shrinks, oncologists then can hopefully re-biopsy the remaining tumor, Nagourney says, "to redouble our efforts in further cytoreduction on the remaining selected clones, and so on."[203]

Besides, if heterogeneity were such a pressing issue, then the many highly correlated results cited elsewhere in this book would not be possible.

I will reiterate the main point: the blind administration of chemotherapy through empirically derived results cannot possibly be better at overcoming the problem of heterogeneity than using the insights gained from modern chemosensitivity assays.

Limitations of the Test

Although the Test is a very good guide to treatment, no single laboratory model can reflect the full complexity of all events taking place in the human body. A model of a bridge is not the same thing as the actual span. The DNA model of the double helix has been seminal to modern biology, but it is not an exact replica of the genetic material that exists in our cells. But science and engineering, while recognizing the limitations of models, also has an urgent need for them.

Researchers at the National Naval Medical Center have put it thus: "There may be a greater potential utility of using DSR [drug sensitivity testing, ed.] to select chemotherapy agents in a clinical situation in which the cancer is more sensitive."[204]

In other words, the test is only as good as the drugs it evaluates. The Test provides crucial evidence on the inherent sensitivity or resistance of cancer cells to various drugs. But it is constrained by the limitations of chemotherapy itself in advanced human cancers. These problems include:

The multiple pathways that cancer cells use to foster their own growth and survival (many of these involving the creation and recruitment of a functioning blood supply[205])

The inherent dose-limiting toxicity of many of the approved agents

The tendency of tumors to develop multiple drug resistance (MDR) to whatever agents are deployed against them.

The Test can choose the best drugs, but its use cannot automatically overcome persistent problems that tend to limit the effectiveness of cytotoxic treatment in general.

IV. TESTING FOR SPECIFIC CANCERS

If randomized controlled trials are generally lacking, what is the evidence for the accuracy (i.e., sensitivity and specificity) of the Test in regard to particular kinds of cancer?

In this section I shall discuss the application of the Test to the chemotherapeutic treatment of specific forms of cancer. The Test is unusual in that its use is not restricted to specific types of cancer (as, for instance, ER and PR receptors or the Oncotype DX™ test are in the main specific to breast cancer). Rather, the Test can be used for virtually every form of cancer from which a fresh and viable tumor specimen can be obtained.‡‡‡

In the following discussion I have been greatly assisted by charts compiled by Robert Nagourney. I have also drawn on various published reports that support the efficacy of the Test in diverse situations.

Breast Cancer

In 2010, in the US there were 209,060 new cases of breast cancer with 40,230 deaths.[206] Chemotherapy routinely figures in the treatment of all but the earliest and least dangerous forms of this disease. For instance, it is commonly used as an adjuvant treatment (after surgery and

---

‡‡‡ In the case of leukemia and other hematological cancers, blood samples can often be used, especially when the patient is in a so-called 'blast crisis.'

radiation) for early-stage breast cancer. It can be used as a 'neoadjuvant' treatment, before surgery, to shrink larger or more difficult tumors and make them more amenable to operation. In later stages of the disease, when the tumor has already metastasized, or spread to other sites, it can be used as a palliative treatment.

Given conventionally, it is not very effective in late-stage disease. According to the NCI, only 3.1 percent of patients treated with systemic chemotherapy for advanced breast cancer were in complete remission for more than five years, and just 1.5 percent remained in remission at 16 years.[207] The challenge for oncologists is to discover which patients are most likely to respond to which drugs.

Breast cancer is unusual in that there is already a certain degree of *personalization* involved in its treatment. In most cases, women are offered the choice of lumpectomy-plus-radiation or the radical Halsted operation.[208] It has been routine for decades to perform assays on preserved tumor samples for estrogen and progesterone receptors, which in turn are used to determine the applicability of certain hormonal therapies. Over the past decade or so it has also become routine to test for an amplification of the HER2-neu gene or an over-expression of its protein product, which shows whether or not the drug trastuzumab (Herceptin) might be beneficial.

More recently oncologists have begun to utilize a genomic panel called Oncotype DX™, which shows whether or not some patients are likely to benefit from adjuvant chemotherapy after surgery. FDA has also approved a blood test called CellSearch, manufactured by Veridex (a subsidiary of Johnson & Johnson) for the detection of circulating tumor cells (CTCs).[209] I do not intend to discuss the utility of these other tests at length. My point is simply that breast cancer is already a disease in which some personalization already takes place.

Breast cancer was also one of the first solid tumors to be treated with chemotherapy. The celebrated Bonadonna regimen (cyclophosphamide + methotrexate + 5-fluorouracil, i.e., CMF) was first announced in the 1970s.[210]

A committee called the Early Breast Cancer Trialists' Collaborative Group (EBCTCG) meets every five years to review data from global breast cancer trials. There is usually a lag time in analyzing and publishing these results, so the latest review (at this writing) dates from 2005, and contains an overview as of the year 2000. This review identified some real benefit to chemotherapy in this situation.

The study involved 28,764 women who participated in 60 trials of combination chemotherapy vs. those who received no chemotherapy. It also included 14,470 women in 17 trials of anthracyclines-containing regimens vs. a CMF-type regimen, and 6,125 women in 11 trials of longer vs. shorter chemotherapy duration. For women who were younger than 50 years of age, chemotherapy reduced their annual relative risk of disease relapse by 37 percent and of death by 30 percent. There was an absolute improvement in 15-year survival of ten percent (from 42 percent to 32 percent).

For women aged 50 to 69 the benefits were smaller. The annual risk of relapse or death from breast cancer was decreased (in relative terms) by 19 percent and the risk of death by 12 percent. This translated into a 3 percent absolute gain in 15-year survival, from 47 percent to 50 percent. (Few women 80 and older were included in the study, and so no conclusions could be reached on this more elderly group.) Because of its date, this study analyzed data before the advent of taxane-containing, dose-dense or trastuzumab-based therapies. Thus, overall results today might be better than are indicated above.

Nonetheless, one of the big problems is that adjuvant chemotherapy is given to almost all women in this situation (especially those who are premenopausal) when, in fact, only a minority of patients are likely to benefit. That is one of the reasons that the Oncotype DX™ test is so desirable—it can eliminate the use of chemotherapy in situations in which it is unlikely to be of any help.

Another way of making the most of chemotherapy, when it is necessary, is to utilize the Test as a decision-making tool. There are, after all, quite a few proposed

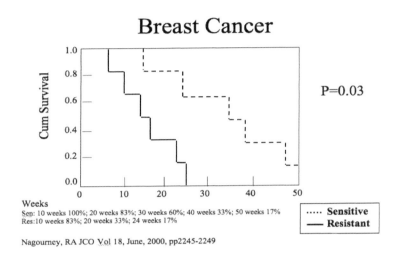

Breast Cancer

P=0.03

Weeks

Sen: 10 weeks 100%; 20 weeks 83%; 30 weeks 60%; 40 weeks 33%; 50 weeks 17%
Res:10 weeks 83%; 20 weeks 33%; 24 weeks 17%

····· **Sensitive**
—— **Resistant**

Nagourney, RA JCO Vol 18, June, 2000, pp2245-2249

regimens for breast cancer, whether in the adjuvant or the palliative setting. And breast cancer was in fact one of the first cancers to be analyzed by the Test, by Speer and Black in the early 1950s.[211]

Nagourney *et al.* published their results on the use of the Test to guide the treatment of breast cancer in the *Journal of Clinical Oncology* in 2000.[212] This was a study of two drugs, gemcitabine + cisplatin, in the treatment of relapsed breast cancer. But buried within the data was an important observation on the effects of this combination when analyzed in the light of the Test.

The above chart graphically demonstrates that re-lapsed breast cancer patients whose cells were resistant to the drugs in question had a worse clinical response than those whose tumors were sensitive to the drugs. These latter patients relapsed and died sooner than those whose tumors were sensitive.

MiCK Assay and Breast Cancer

At the 2009 ASCO meeting, DiaTech scientists presented a paper on the chemosensitivity of patients with breast cancer. They showed how sensitivity correlated with prior chemotherapy and explained the implications of this for personalized treatment planning.[213]

In this study, 57 live tumor samples were sent to their Montreal laboratory and apoptosis was measured over 48 hours with various drugs. These laboratory results were then compared to the clinical status of the patient. (In this blinded experiment, doctors gave chemotherapy without knowing the outcome of the test.)

The authors found that MiCK could be used to evalu-ate susceptibility to chemotherapy of the breast cancer cells of individual patients. After being subjected to che-motherapy, breast cancer cells showed altered chemosen-sitivity profiles, with persistent sensitivity to some drugs, but reduced sensitivity to others. They concluded that these data "may be useful to MDs in selecting chemother-apy for individual patients. MiCK may also be useful in developing new drugs and new combination therapies."[214]

In South Korea a group using an adenosine triphosphate (ATP)-based chemotherapy response assay also reported excellent results using this test in breast cancer. According to them, it has the advantage of standardization, evaluability, reproducibility and accuracy, and can be performed on relatively small numbers of tumor cells.[215]

A total of 43 patients were enrolled in a study published in the journal *Breast* in 2008. Chemosensitivity tests were successfully performed in 40 of these patients, or 93 percent. Half of these 40 patients received neoadjuvant or adjuvant chemotherapy for metastatic breast cancer. The chemotherapy regimens used were doxorubicin + docetaxel or doxorubicin + paclitaxel. The mean cell death rate was lower in non-responders than in those who responded to therapy.

Table 2

ATP-based Assay for Breast Cancer

	Sensitivity	Specificity	Positive Predictive Value	Negative Predictive Value	Diagnostic Accuracy
the Test	78.6%	100%	100%	66.7%	85%

Data: Kim 2008

Once again I will point out that the diagnostic accuracy of the standard tests for estrogen receptors (ER) and progesterone receptors (PR) were lower than that achieved using this form of the Test. Yet health insurers around the world routinely pay for ER and PR tests but not for the Test.

Also important was the Korean group's finding that various genetic markers were *not* significantly associated with the patients' response to chemotherapy. This included expressions of various genes (p53, erb-B2, Ki67, Bcl-2, Bcl-xL, and annexin I).[216] Without going into detail, this demonstrates that whatever the current excitement over genomic testing, results can be more predictive when one brings actual cancer cells together with drugs *in vitro* before choosing treatment.

Ovarian Cancer

In 2010, there were 21,880 new cases of ovarian cancer in the US, with 13,850 deaths.[217] Some stage I patients may not need chemotherapy. But chemotherapy is routinely used in the treatment of high-risk stage I epithelial cancer of the ovaries, as well as most other stages of the disease.

Almost all regimens for ovarian cancer include the drug cisplatin. It has been known for a long time that the mineral platinum has a destructive effect on the generative organs. In his *Materia Medica*, the homeopath Willis A. Dewey, MD (1858-1938) mentioned platinum as causing "early and profuse menses of dark clotted blood, accompanied by bearing down pains; the ovaries are sensitive and have burning pains in them."[218]

Some decades later, platinum's anticancer effects were discovered serendipitously in the course of studies on electrolysis using a platinum electrode. Barnett Rosenberg of the University of Michigan first used this mineral in cancer experiments in the 1960s.[219] Some patients'

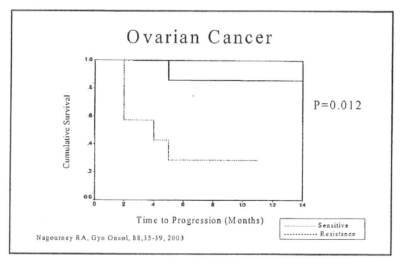

cells, however, are resistant to platinum, although few of them know that when beginning treatment. Since platinum drugs can be very toxic, it would be highly desirable to check this with the Test before initiating treatment.

In 2003, Nagourney published a study on 27 ovarian cancer patients.[220] Of these, there were 7 complete responses and 12 partial responses, for an overall response rate of 70 percent. "*Ex vivo* [the Test, ed.] results correlated with response, time to progression, and survival, remaining significant when adjusted for platinum-resistance and number of prior therapies," he reported. "The results of the *ex vivo* analyses correlate with clinical outcomes."[221]

ChemoFX and Ovarian Cancer

In 2006, scientists at the Precision Therapeutics laboratory in Pittsburgh published the results of using their proprietary ChemoFx™ form of the Test to guide the treatment of ovarian cancer.[222] The main endpoint was the progression-free interval (PFI). There was a statistically significant correlation between the assay's prediction of response and PFI in 256 cases, with an exact or partial match between drug(s) assayed and those received.

The median PFI for patients treated with drugs that were assayed as resistant was 9 months, but was 14 months for those with drugs assayed as intermediately sensitive. The median PFI had not yet been achieved for those with drugs assayed as sensitive. (In other words, some patients still had not progressed.)

The authors concluded:

"These data indicate that the ChemoFx assay is predictive of PFI in ovarian cancer. As the majority of ovarian cancers display different degrees of response to different chemotherapy agents *ex vivo*, the incorporation of assay information into treatment selection has the potential to improve clinical outcomes in ovarian cancer patients."[223]

Similarly, a randomized trial in the UK using an ATP-based chemosensitivity test also showed positive results. Ninety-four of 180 patients were randomized to receive assay-directed therapy, while 86 received chemotherapy by their physician's choice. Median follow-up time for analysis was 18 months. A response was assessable in 147 patients: 40.5 percent achieved a partial or complete response in the chemosensitivity-directed group vs. 31.5 percent in the physician's-choice group. This represented a 28.6 percent increase in responses.

Twelve of 39 (41 percent) of patients who crossed over from the physician's-choice arm then obtained a response. Overall survival differences were not statistically significant, probably because of the relatively small size of the trial.

"This small randomized clinical trial has documented a trend towards improved response and progression-free survival for assay-directed treatment," the authors wrote.[224]

In February 2010, the National Comprehensive Cancer Network® (NCCN) updated its clinical practice guidelines for oncology (NCCN Guidelines™) for ovarian cancer including fallopian tube cancer and primary peritoneal cancer to include the use of the Test as part of its 'Principles of Chemotherapy' section.

While the revised NCCN Guidelines state that this technology is not intended to supplant standard-of-care chemotherapy, the Test is being used at some NCCN Member Institutions for decisions related to future chemotherapy "in situations where there are multiple equivalent chemotherapy options available."[225]

This is an NCCN category 3 recommendation, meaning that the current level of evidence is not sufficient to supplant standard-of-care chemotherapy. Nonetheless, it represented a small "foot in the door" victory for the Test.

As Karen Kaplan, CEO of the Ovarian Cancer National Alliance, commented:

"We offer our gratitude to NCCN on behalf of the many ovarian cancer patients who could be faced with the potential side effects of ineffective chemotherapies. Not only are oncologists recognizing the benefits of using chemosensitivity and resistance assays when faced with equivalent therapeutic options, but they are also paving the way for greater support of personalized medicine in oncology."[226]

The Loizzi Study

The purpose of this study, performed at the University of California, Irvine (UCI) was to determine the outcomes in patients who had recurrent ovarian carcinoma after extreme drug resistance assay-directed therapy. This is the type of assay employed by Oncotech, which is now part of Exiqon, Inc.

Table 3
Retrospective Study of Response and Survival
in Recurrent Ovarian Cancer

	Overall response rate	Median overall survival	Median progression-free survival
Empiric treatment	35%	21 month	7 months
Assay guided platinum sensitive	65%	38 months	15 months
Improvement		81%	114.3%

Data from Loizzi, 2003

Fifty women were treated with chemotherapy that was guided by an extreme drug resistance assay. They were compared with 50 well-matched control subjects who were treated empirically. "In the platinum-sensitive group, patients with extreme drug resistance-directed therapy had an overall response rate of 65 percent compared with 35 percent in the patients who were treated empirically," the Irvine authors wrote.

The overall survival was 38 months and the progression-free median survival was 15 months in the extreme drug resistance assay group compared with 21 and 7 months in the control group, respectively, differences which were statistically significant. However, in the platinum-resistant group, there was no improved outcome in the patients who underwent assay-guided therapy.

The authors concluded:

"Our results indicate an improved outcome in patients with recurrent ovarian carcinoma who have platinum sensitive disease and who underwent extreme drug resistance-directed chemotherapy."[227]

Portsmouth RCT of Ovarian Cancer

There has been one RCT of the Test in the case of ovarian cancer, conducted by Ian A. Cree, MD *et al.* at Queen Alexandra Hospital in Portsmouth, England.

The primary aim was to compare the response and progression-free survival rates in women who had platinum-resistant and recurrent ovarian cancer. Some were treated according to an ATP-based version of the Test, while others were treated by the physician's choice of drugs. A total of 180 patients were randomized, with 94 getting chemotherapy directed by the Test and 86 getting physician's choice chemotherapy. The median follow-up time at analysis was 18 months. Response was assessable in 147 of the 180 patients (Table 4).

Table 4
Ovarian Cancer RCT of Physician's Choice
vs. the Test (ATP-based)

	Clinical Response Rate (CR + PR)	CRR by intent-to-treat analysis	PFS by intent-to-treat analysis
Physicians' Choice	31.5%	26%	93
ATP test	40.5%	31%	104
Percent increase	28.6%	19.2%	11.8%

Data from Cree, *Anticancer Drugs.* 2007;18:1093-1101

Although no difference was seen in overall survival between the groups, 12 out of 39 (or 30.7 percent) of patients who crossed over from the physician's-choice arm then obtained a response with the Test. The failure to detect a difference in overall survival may have been due to the fact that the trial was 'underpowered' (i.e., it had too few participants to detect this effect in such an advanced patient population).[228]

Ovarian Cancer (MiCK Assay)

In 2010, DiaTech Oncology reported at the American Society of Clinical Oncology (ASCO) annual meeting on results of a clinical trial in ovarian cancer.[229] The test was able to predict both increased response and survival for ovarian cancer.

The results showed increased overall survival in 92 percent of patients who received their drugs based on the MiCK version of the Test, compared to only 76 percent of those who received treatment that was not recommended by the test.

There was also a significantly higher overall response rate (82 vs. 54 percent) in the MiCK-guided patients. Stage III and IV ovarian cancer patients had significantly increased survival rates (94 vs. 77 percent alive at 24 months). The clinical benefit rate was 85 percent for patients who received drugs that were highly active in the assay, compared to only 57 percent for patients receiving less active forms of chemotherapy.

The test pointed to several ways that insurers could save money by doing the test. Thus, single drug therapy produced better results than combination chemotherapy in approximately 30 percent of patients. Less expensive generic drugs were at least equally effective compared to more expensive drugs in 75 percent of patients.

"The impressive and statistically significant survival and response data in this study show that the DiaTech MiCK assay can be an effective tool for oncologists in determining the best chemotherapy treatment for a cancer patient," said Dr. Emery Salom, Chief Dept of OB/GYN Palmetto General Hospital, Assistant Professor Florida International University, Herbert Wertheim College of Medicine.

"It is also important to note the data provided guidance on generic drug use and single vs combination therapies," said Dr. Cary Presant, Medical Director DiaTech Oncology, Professor of Medicine, University of Southern California. "This is good news for ovarian cancer patients and is clearly a major step to provide more effective personalized care, and often less expensive and less toxic treatment of cancer patients."[230]

Endometrial Cancer (MiCK Assay)

In 2010, the MiCK assay was also tested for its effects in endometrial cancer.[231] All specimens from hysterectomies were processed by DiaTech's laboratory, where single cells were suspended in individual wells. The combination of doxorubicin, cisplatin and paclitaxel was tested as well as paclitaxel, carboplatin, doxorubicin, cisplatin, ifosfamide, and vincristine as single drugs.

Apoptosis (i.e., programmed cell death) was then continuously measured for 48 hours. Fifteen of nineteen patients (78.9 percent) had successful assays. The highest mean chemosensitivity was seen with the combination of cisplatin, doxorubicin and paclitaxel. The lowest mean sensitivity was seen with the individual agents carboplatin and paclitaxel. This will come as no surprise to oncologists.

However, the significant finding was that in 25 percent of patients one of the single drugs had higher chemosensitivity than combination chemotherapy. Thus, although on average the standard recommendation was warranted, in a quarter of the cases a single agent was better than the combination and significantly less toxic.

Non-Small Cell Lung Cancer

There are several published abstracts on the use of Nagourney's form of the Test (called the EVA-PCD™ assay) to choose targeted or anti-angiogenic agents for treating non-small cell lung cancer. Although these studies involve relatively few patients, they are suggestive of what might be attained with more wide-scale use.

First a word about targeted agents. Various types of targeted therapies exist, but most attention has been paid to those that target angiogenesis. These are small molecules that attach to and shut off various pathways by which tumors promote the growth of blood vessels. According to the theory of the late Harvard Medical School professor Judah Folkman, MD, tumors are compelled either to grow new blood vessels or recruit established ones in order to fulfill their many nutritional requirements (primarily for glucose). Without a well-functioning blood supply, tumors will remain about the size of a pencil point.[232]

The FDA has already approved eight anti-angiogenic drugs,[233] and dozens more are in the pipeline.[234] Thus, selecting from a growing list of targeted agents has become a difficult problem.

The entry of targeted agents has already demanded a certain degree of customized medicine. That is because there are several known prognostic and predictive factors,§§§ but these involve various complex and overlapping cell surface markers.

To complicate matters, most of these targeted agents are extremely expensive. Avastin alone costs $90,000 per year (although the manufacturer, Genentech, caps the annual cost at $55,000 for people earning less than $100,000 per year).[235] Because of the uncertainty of getting a response, many doctors rule out the use of a drug that might be dramatically effective in only a small minority of patients.

To overcome these problems, Nagourney *et al.* applied the Test to cells of patients with NSCLC, using only drugs that were approved by FDA for that indication. Twenty-five patients were enrolled, of whom 22 were evaluable. One patient had a stroke before he could begin treatment, while two had inadequate progression-free survival (PFS) at the time of treatment (Table 5).

---

§§§ E.g., ERCC1, RRM1/2 and EGFR mutations

Table 5
Outcome in NSCLC Using Nagourney's Test

	No.	CR	PR	SD	PD	OR	CB
Test guided	22	2	10	9	1	12	21
RR	----	9%	45%	41%	5%	54%	95%

Data from Nagourney, 2009
RR = Response Rate,
CR= Complete response,
PR = Partial response, PD = Progressive disease,
OR = Overall response, CB = Clinical benefit.

The "ex vivo best regimens" (EVBRs), chosen based on Nagourney's form of the Test, were as follows:
• 10/25 or 40% of patients received cisplatin (CDDP) plus Gemzar (gemcitabine)
• 7/25 or 28% received cisplatin plus a taxane-based drug
• 5/25 or 20% received erlotinib (Tarceva)
• 1/25 or 4% received cisplatin plus vinorelbine
• 1/25 or 4% received cisplatin plus irinotecan
• 1/25 or 4% received Ifex plus gemcitabine

Perhaps equally impressive was the fact that 6 of the 22 stage IV patients who were evaluated were 'converted' into good candidates for surgery or radiation therapy because of this therapy. They then had the potential for long-term survival or even cure that this implies. Accrual into this study continues, but the time to progression

(TTP) as of June 2009 ranged from a low of 1.2 to a high of 35+ months. The overall survival ranges from 1.7 to 46+ months.[236]

Obviously, this was not a randomized study, so we do not have an exact idea of how patients would have fared had they used some other method of choosing their drugs. But we have seen how patients fared in conventional clinical trials. For instance, in one trial (analyzed below) the median progression free survival (PFS) was just *6.1 months* for the group that received cisplatin + gemcitabine (CG) plus placebo vs. *6.5 months* in those who received either low-dose or high-dose Avastin (bevacizumab).

Similarly, in a 2010 randomized trial, from Emory University, carboplatin + paclitaxel was given to one half of the patients. These patients had a 12.5 percent overall response rate (ORR).[237,****] Meanwhile, when NSCLC treatment was directed by the Test, as in the above Nagourney study, the ORR was 54 percent, more than four times as great!

What was the main difference? Primarily that in the Emory clinical trial the same drugs were given to all patients in the standard therapy arm of the study.

**** Those who also got an experimental medicine, vorinostat, did somewhat better.

In the second case, however, drugs were chosen to match the reactions of cancer cells brought into direct physical contact for 72 hours with candidate drugs under laboratory conditions.

Since 40 percent of the patients received the doublet of gemcitabine and cisplatin some might think that this fact alone was responsible for the superior results. One might argue that this is an especially potent combination.

However, in a December 2009 Japanese trial of this doublet 45 patients were enrolled, and all of them were assessable for response and toxicity. None had a complete response and the partial response rate was 37.8 percent.[238] This was much better than for carboplatin + paclitaxel, but it still hardly compares to the 54 percent ORR achieved with therapy guided by the Test. In the latter case, the choice of this doublet did not come about because of intuition on the part of an oncologist, but because the measurement of living and dying cancer cells directed their use. Comparison with this Japanese study points to the huge potential when drugs are chosen rationally before they are put into the body of a human being.

Small Cell Lung Cancer

Small cell lung cancer (SCLC) is a less common form of the disease than its non-small cell counterpart, representing about 15 percent of all cases.

Chemotherapy routinely improves the survival of patients with both limited-stage or extensive-stage small cell lung cancer (SCLC). However, according to the National Cancer Institute (NCI), it is curative in only a minority of such patients.

Because patients who have SCLC also tend to develop distant metastases, localized forms of treatment, such as surgical resection or radiation therapy, rarely result in long-term survival or cure. By including chemotherapy in the overall treatment program, however, survival can be somewhat prolonged.

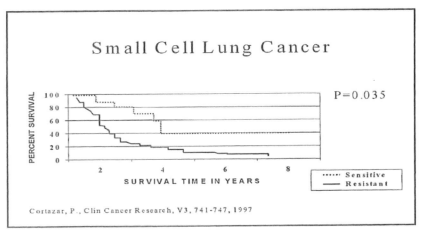

There is generally a four to five-fold improvement in the median survival compared to patients who are given no chemotherapy.[239] The most widely used standard regimen is the doublet of platinum and etoposide. So far, no consistent survival benefit has resulted from increasing dose intensity or density, by altering the mode of administration or by maintenance chemotherapy.

However, there have already been promising results in the treatment of small cell lung cancer guided by chemosensitivity testing.

Patricia Cortazar, MD, then of the National Naval Medical Center, Bethesda, showed the benefit of using the Test to determine treatment in SCLC.[240] In 1997, 54 patients with previously untreated SCLC were given four cycles of the standard doublet of etoposide + cisplatin, along with concurrent radiotherapy. This was followed by four cycles of additional chemotherapy with drugs chosen via the Test.

Here are the author's conclusions:

"The median actuarial survival of 8 patients treated with their IVBR [*in vitro* Best Regimen, ed.] was 38.5 months compared to 19 months for the 46 patients treated with empiric chemotherapy. Selection of individualized chemotherapy regimens is labor intensive but feasible in limited-stage SCLC. Treatment with an individualized IVBR in our patients was associated with *prolonged patient survival*..."[241] (emphasis added).

Thus, on average, SCLC patients whose adjuvant treatment was guided by the Test lived *twice as long* as those whose treatment was based on the results of RCTs.

Malignant Melanoma

Superficial malignant melanoma can be cured by surgery if it is caught in the early stages. In addition, melanoma is one type of cancer that is somewhat responsive to immunological controls, and new treatments, including melanoma vaccines, are frequently proposed.[242] However, the generally refractory nature of this disease to standard drugs makes it "potentially a candidate for treatment with different classes of agents, including experimental therapies."[243]

As a review written by researchers from the H. Lee Moffitt Cancer Center in Florida put it, regional techniques provide the greatest control and have minimal operative morbidity. Until new regimens are available, systemic therapy continues to be associated with considerable toxicity and only marginal response rates.[244]

The empiric chemotherapy agent of choice is dacarbazine (DTIC), but response rates using this drug are only in the region of 15 to 25 percent, with a median duration of response of around five to six months. Only one to two percent of all patients treated with dacarbazine experience a complete long-term response

In an attempt to improve the generally poor results with chemotherapy there have been many trials of multiagent regimens involving the drugs cisplatin, carmustine, tamoxifen, vinblastine, and BCNU given alongside dacarbazine, but none has yet shown significantly bazine, but none has yet shown significantly improved results over dacarbazine alone.

Similarly, regimens employing multi-agent chemotherapy plus immune-modulating cytokines (INF-a2b, interleukin-2) have not yielded improved results over simple dacarbazine therapy, although the University of Texas M.D. Anderson Cancer Center, in Houston, has reported complete response rates of 20 percent and long-term survival in about 10 percent of cases using a chemotherapy regime of cisplatin, vinblastine and dacarbazine

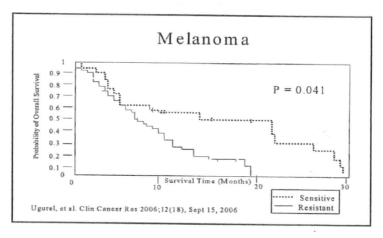

in combination with both IFN-a2b and IL-2.[245]

Selma Ugurel, MD, *et al.* published a study on the use of the Test in melanoma in *Clinical Cancer Research* in September 2006. This trial showed a dramatic difference in the survival of patients whose cells were sensitive to particular drugs compared to those whose cells were resistant. This trial of the Dermatologic

Cooperative Oncology Group was based at the German Cancer Research Center, Heidelberg, which is the largest biomedical research institute in Germany.

The authors enrolled 82 patients and gave assay-directed chemotherapy to 57 of these; 53 were available for analysis for objective response, safety, overall survival and progression-free survival. Forty-two percent of the patients were found to be chemosensitive, while the remainder had cells that were resistant on the Test.

Table 6
Response Rates and Survival in
Malignant Melanoma Patients

	Objective response	Progression arrest (PR+CR+SD)	Overall survival
Resistant (58% cases)	16.1%	22.6%	7.4 mos.
Sensitive (42% cases)	36.4%	59.1%	14.6 mos.
Percentage increase	126%	161.5%	97.3%

Data from Ugurel, *et al.*, 2006

As a general rule, patients whose tumor cells were sensitive to various forms of chemotherapy had response rates and survival time approximately double that of patients whose cells were resistant. Objective responses were also more than double in the group found to be sensitive, as was the overall category of progression arrest.

Overall survival was also nearly double. These results are summarized in Table 6, above.

Chronic Lymphocytic Leukemia

Leukemia is the name given to a broad category of cancers that start in the blood-forming tissue such as the bone marrow and causes large numbers of blood cells to be produced and enter the bloodstream. The total number of new leukemia cases in the United States in 2010 was 43,050 and there were 21,840 deaths.

Chronic lymphocytic leukemia (CLL) is the most common form of leukemia in North America. There are about 1.8 to 3 cases per 100,000 of the general population, but the incidence increases to 30.5 per 100,000 in people between the ages of 80 and 84. CLL affects more males than females, and has therefore historically been thought of as a disease of elderly men. For reasons no one fully understands, this disease is far less common in Asia than it is in North America and Europe.

Not long ago, chronic leukemia was considered untreatable. "One should do nothing that threatens to ...lessen the comfort of the patient in such cases," was the sage advice of a prewar encyclopedia of cancer.[246] While impressive progress has been made in the treatment of certain types of leukemia, these advances are most dramatic in the treatment of childhood leukemia, which are almost always of the acute type. Progress in the treatment of chronic leukemia has not been quite as rapid, but even so there have been some hopeful developments in the past few years.

Since the mid-1950s the standard treatment for more aggressive forms of the disease has been chlorambucil (Leukeran). This agent, taken orally, is rapidly absorbed into the bloodstream. Since the 1980s, though, a new class of drugs has been used in CLL.

These are called the purine analogs, and include fludarabine monophosphate (Fludara) and 2-CDA (cladribine). Fludarabine is the drug most commonly used when patients no longer respond to chlorambucil. Another drug of the monoclonal antibody type, Rituxan (rituximab), has also proven to be extremely useful.

There have been some dramatic results when the Test was used to predict the effect of drugs in chronic lympho-

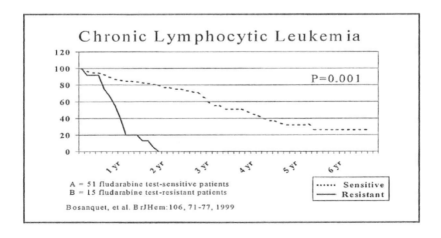

Chronic Lymphocytic Leukemia

P=0.001

A = 51 fludarabine test-sensitive patients
B = 15 fludarabine test-resistant patients

...... Sensitive
—— Resistant

Bosanquet, et al. B rJHem:106, 71-77, 1999

cytic leukemia (CLL).[247]

Andrew G. Bosanquet, MD, and colleagues used the Test for several decades at the Royal United Hospital in Bath, England. They studied 66 patients with chronic lymphocytic leukemia (CLL). Fifty-one were found to be sensitive to the drug fludarabine. Another fifteen were resistant.[248]

The decision of whether to use fludarabine (Fludara) or the earlier drug chlorambucil is an important one, both therapeutically and economically. Fludarabine is about 40 times as expensive as chlorambucil.[249] It is also sometimes associated with intense toxicity. According to the manufacturer, the drug can cause "severe central nervous system toxicity, including coma, seizures, agitation and confusion...."[250]

So if there were a way to identify those patients who were *not* likely to benefit from this drug, that alone "could advance disease management both clinically and financially," said Bosanquet.[251]

The authors first used the Test to determine whether or not patients' cancer cells were either sensitive or resistant to fludarabine. When the test indicated that patients were indeed sensitive to fludarabine they responded clinically to the drug 69 percent of the time and their overall median survival was 41.7 months. But when the test showed that they were resistant, only 7 percent responded and their median survival time was 7.9 months. Thus, *patients with sensitive cells lived more than five times longer* than those with resistant cells.

Table 7 summarizes the results.

Table 7

Correlation of the Test (DiSC) Results with Response Rate and Overall Survival In Chronic Lymphocytic Leukemia

DiSC Test Results	Response rate	Overall median survival
Fludarabine resistant cells	7%	7.9
Fludarabine sensitive cells	69%	41.7
Percentage increase	885.7%	427.8%

Data from Bosanquet, *et al.*, 1999

The authors reasonably concluded that not all CLL patients should receive fludarabine. The results of the Test were a "powerful independent prognostic factor" in deciding whether or not patients would respond.

For the patients whose cancer cells were resistant to this drug, however effective it might be in other peoples' cases, there was no justification for administering it.

"Disease management, response, survival and use of financial resources might be significantly improved if therapy choice in CLL patients was guided by DiSC assay," the authors stated.[252]

Yet, a decade later, this has not happened and in fact Andrew Bosanquet's laboratory in Bath, which provided the Test in Great Britain, closed its doors in 2009 for lack of financial support.[253]

According to the National Comprehensive Cancer Network (NCCN) "fludarabine is the foundation of active regimens for both untreated and heavily pretreated patients."[254] There is no mention of pre-testing these patients' cells to see if the patients are likely to respond to the drug.

In fact, as things currently stand, virtually all CLL patients who have the means are likely to receive fludarabine at some point in their treatment, without their doctors pre-testing their cells to see where they fall in the drug-sensitivity scale.

This is great news for Bayer HealthCare Pharmaceuticals Inc., which markets fludarabine as Fludara, and in 2008 earned 100 million Euros ($150 million USD at the time) in worldwide sales.[255]

But this one-size-fits-all philosophy leads to a great deal of unnecessary treatment with a potentially toxic drug, as well as lost opportunities to utilize other more effective drugs.

the Test could reduce the social cost of administering Fludara, while at the same time focusing use on the drug on just those patients who are likely to benefit.

Pediatric ALL

Pediatric acute lymphocytic leukemia (ALL) is a disease in which chemotherapy is notably successful. But Nagourney *et al.* showed a remarkable difference in survival between those who cells were resistant to chemotherapy and those whose cells were sensitive.

In a 1991 paper in the *Lancet*, Bosanquet also showed that no patient with hematological (blood-based) cancer whose cells showed extreme drug resistance in the Test responded to chemotherapy. As the *in vitro* test response rate increased, so did the clinical response rate of the

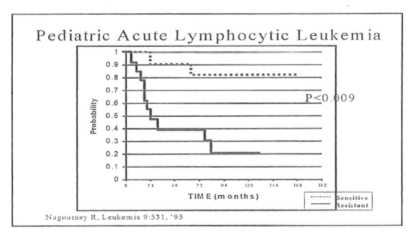

Nagourney R, Leukemia 9:531, '95

patients themselves. Patients who used drugs that worked in the laboratory also had longer survival.[256]

Adult Brain Cancer

In 2010, there were an estimated 22,020 new cases of brain and other nervous system tumors in the US with 13,140 deaths. Brain tumors constitute 85 to 90 percent of all the primary central nervous system (CNS) tumors. Worldwide, approximately 176,000 new cases of brain and other CNS tumors were diagnosed in 2000, and approximately 128,000 died.[257]

Chemotherapy (such as temozolomide, Temodor®) is rarely the mainstay treatment, but it is frequently used as part of a multi-modal therapy, as it may help prolong survival in some tumor types. For instance, it has been reported to lengthen disease-free survival in patients with gliomas, medulloblastoma, and some germ cell tumors.[258] Chemotherapy is also used in most patients who have leptomeningeal involvement (from a primary or a metastatic tumor) as well as tumors in the cerebrospinal fluid.

There are promising studies on the use of the Test in brain tumors. For instance, in Guangzhou, China, scientists used the Test as well as a marker for resistance (the repair protein MGMT) to evaluate the efficacy of individualized chemotherapy. The patients in question all had confirmed malignant gliomas and were treated between 2001 and 2006 at Sun Yat Sen University in that city. Fresh tumor tissue obtained during the operation was immediately sent for the Test using the MTT assay (a modern-day version of the old tetrazolium test).[259] After radiation therapy, the patients received chemotherapy according to the results of their individualized Test results.

Overall, 49 cases were evaluable. Of these, 6 (12 percent) achieved complete remission, 10 (20 percent) achieved partial remission, 20 (41 percent) had stable disease and 13 (27 percent) progressed. The objective response rate was 33 percent and the disease control rate was 73 percent. J.P. Zhang and his colleagues concluded: "Individualized chemotherapy ...for patients with malignant gliomas" using the Test "could improve overall response rate."[260]

Comments on the Clinical Data

The above results provide a broad overview of what can be achieved with the use of the Test. Obviously, we are not talking about a miraculous magic bullet—chemotherapy has intrinsic limitations—but a way of squeezing the greatest potential benefit out of the various drugs and drug combinations that already exist. The Test can also be used to evaluate complementary and alternative products, as well as anti-angiogenic agents.

As the reader reviews the above studies he or she may wonder how oncologists can continue to claim that the Test has not been proven effective at choosing the best treatments for individual patients. One comes across various arguments, such as that the tests are cumbersome, time consuming, inaccurate or too expensive to perform on a routine basis. Some of these criticisms may have been justified in regard to earlier incarnations of the

Test, such as the clonogenic assay. But this sort of criticism typically fails to differentiate between the older assays and the newer tests that are based on the detection of programmed cell death (PCD) in fresh cells.

The current apoptosis-based tests can usually be performed within one week. This is enough time to allow physicians and patients both to utilize the data to reach a decision on chemotherapy.

What about the cost? At most chemosensitivity testing laboratories it ranges from $2,500 to $3,500, depending on the extent of the testing. This is not an extraordinary charge, considering the value of the information that is provided. In an era in which a single chemotherapeutic drug (Folotyn™) can cost as much as $30,000 per month, it makes economic as well as medical sense to find out in advance what is likely to work and what is not.[261]

The nub of the problem is that medical insurance plans often will not pay for the Test.†††† And so patients must largely foot the bill themselves. The essential financial problem, then, is not the cost of the procedure itself but the misguided policies of the health insurance

---

†††† Weisenthal once wrote that Medicare paid $620 as their share of his testing. However, he recently told me that Medicare policy varies geographically. In Pennsylvania, for instance, reimbursement is considerably higher, while in most jurisdictions the Test is not a covered service.

companies and agencies (such as Medicare, Blue Cross, etc.) that refuse to pay for this cost-effective test.

There is evidence that wide-scale adoption of the Test would help not just patients, but consumers and insurance companies as well. In June 2009, DiaTech Oncology presented a paper on this topic at the annual meeting of the American Society for Clinical Oncology (ASCO).[262]

They studied the claims for lung, breast, colon or ovarian cancer patients among the 48,927 employees of a large self-insured corporation. There were 196 patients who developed these forms of cancer during a 3.5-year period. The total treatment cost was $5,647,165, of which the cost of anticancer drugs was $1,149,404. But when only drugs that were active in their proprietary form of the Test, the MiCK assay, were used the average savings were impressive.

Treatment via this form of the Test "could save a high percentage" of chemotherapy costs, as well as a "substantial percentage of overall costs" of cancer care for such organizations, the authors reported.[263] These savings varied from 9.9 percent to 62.7 percent depending on effectiveness and duration of the treatment for different types and stages of cancer. But the true economic value of treatment that is guided by the Test would be higher, since use of active chemotherapy could "increase quality of life and employment, and reduce disability and side effects."[264]

This paper shows the huge cost savings that the Test potentially represents. The allegedly excessive up-front costs appear burdensome, but are actually economical in the long run.

V. THE ASCO REVIEW

As I have shown, the 1983 by Selby, Buick and Tannock in the *New England Journal of Medicine* was a major blow to the acceptance of the Test. Even more damaging were a pair of reviews published in the *Journal of Clinical Oncology* (JCO) in September 2004.[265] In fact, these articles signaled the end of any further studies of the topic by NCI or other influential or powerful groups within oncology. It is a blow from which the field has yet to recover.

After some preliminary success in gaining acceptance from the insurance industry in California,[266] it seemed as if the Test were poised for acceptance nationwide. But rather than getting the green light that they anticipated, leaders of the chemosensitivity field were shocked to learn that their method was being condemned in a blatantly prejudicial manner.

How did this disastrous 2004 ASCO review come about? At the time that ASCO decided to examine the issue, the Blue Cross and Blue Shield Association Technology Evaluation Center (TEC) was already conducting a systematic review of the Test under contract to the Health Care Financing Administration (HCFA).

The two reviews became intertwined when ASCO was granted access to a draft of the TEC report. It independently reviewed the articles selected for inclusion in TEC review but used the latter as its template. The TEC review, whose first author was David J. Samson, was eventually published in the same issue of the *Journal of Clinical Oncology* as the ASCO review.[267] The first author of the ASCO review was Deborah Schrag, MD, then of Memorial Sloan-Kettering Cancer Center (MKSCC), New York.

Schrag and Samson's reports are often cited and analyzed in tandem and in essence they are part of the same review process. For the sake of simplicity, therefore, I will deal with both the "Schrag" and "Samson" evaluations collectively as the "ASCO review," although technically speaking there were two reviews with slightly different perspectives.

With TEC's help, the ASCO Working Group compiled a database on the topic of the Test, which grew to include 1,139 abstracts from 1966 to January 2004 (a testimony to the depth of research on this topic). Out of this large amount of data, however, they eventually selected just 12 articles for review. There were technical reasons for choosing just these particular papers and as we shall see, this stringent selection process eventually led to a serious bias.

First of all, they deliberately and systematically excluded all the correlations that are the main proof of the effectiveness of the Test. They were only interested in papers that compared *survival rates* in patients treated under chemosensitivity guidance *vs. those treated by the empiric method.*

In their zeal to cover the most prominent forms of the Test, they took what they felt was a representative sample of papers, of past techniques as well as present. There were several individuals on the panel who had been closely associated in the past with the outdated clonogenic assay. Perhaps in deference to them, the clonogenic assay was put on an equal footing in this study with more modern forms of the Test.

This would be like conducting an overall review of the value of radiotherapy that focused critical attention on the results achieved with outdated cobalt machines from the 1930s and 1940s, but then failed to appreciate the revolution represented by intensity modulated radiotherapy. Negative conclusions from such a review would be meaningless. Given this methodology, the ASCO reviewers not surprisingly reached negative overall conclusions:

"Review of the literature [particularly these dozen articles, ed.] does not identify any CSRAs [chemosensitivity and resistance assays, ed.] for which the evidence base is sufficient to support use in oncology practice."[268]

Considering the centrality of the ASCO review to the present-day wide-scale rejection of the Test, it is important to go over this article in some detail, with an emphasis on the faulty reasoning that led to these incorrect conclusions.

Flaws in the ASCO Argument

There are deep flaws in the 2004 ASCO review, so many that I find it shocking that an organization of ASCO's stature would lend its name and prestige to such a statement.

The 2004 ASCO review began with faint praise for the general concept of the Test. "There is an intrinsic appeal," the authors wrote, to the notion of "using effective agents while sparing unnecessary ones."[269] That said, they then rejected all current implementation of chemosensitivity and resistance testing.

As noted, the most important thing to realize is that the majority of the Working Group's time and effort was taken up evaluating *old and outdated assays*. Perhaps this was not surprising, since, as I have said, a senior member of the panel was Daniel D. Von Hoff, MD, Sydney Salmon's protege and himself a one-time vocal proponent of the outdated clonogenic assay. Another panel member was Anne Hamburger, who co-authored Salmon's original paper in the *NEJM* on the clonogenic assay.[270]

"It is difficult for anyone to determine why oncologists have not paid more attention to the use of *in vitro* predictive tests in the care of their patients," Von Hoff wrote in 1990.[271] Yet in 2004 he co-authored this ASCO report, which did more damage to this field than anything that had preceded it.

In the interim, it might be worth noting, Dr. Von Hoff had become, among other things, Chief Scientific Officer of US Oncology, "one of the nation's largest research networks specializing in Phase I-IV oncology clinical trials."[272] He is as heavily involved with the conduct of clinical trials, including RCTs, as almost anyone else in the country.‡‡‡‡ One reason for this change in emphasis can be gauged by a revealing anecdote he related in a 1990 paper in *the Journal of the National Cancer Institute (JNCI):*

"At a recent meeting in New York, as I was placing my slides in a carousel, I heard someone in the audience say, 'He's not going to talk about *in vitro* predictive assays again, is he?' I turned around and said, 'No, you don't have to worry about that, I will be talking about new drugs.' However, it drove home a point....[N]o one wants to hear about *in vitro* predictive assays."[273]

Not surprisingly, in recent years, few if any of his papers concerns this sort of assay.

---

‡‡‡‡ At this writing, Von Hoff has had 112 PubMed listed articles in the clinical trial category alone. By contrast, the distinguished president of the University of Texas MD Anderson Cancer Center, John Mendelsohn, MD, has just seven.

As UC Irvine Prof. John Fruehauf and University of Arizona Cancer Center President David S. Alberts§§§§ (another Sydney Salmon protege) have pointed out, the majority of citations offered in the ASCO review were "significantly flawed and of only historical interest. Clonogenic assays, which comprised three of the 12 papers, have long been known to be fraught with various technical problems, and are no longer offered on a commercial basis."[274]

Some of the other forms of the Test included in the study were also defunct by the time of the ASCO review. Fruehauf and Alberts pointed out that three of the forms of the Test analyzed were not offered nationally on a commercial basis. "Fortunately, technology has moved on,"[275] they added.

But the ASCO committee emphatically did not move on, but included outdated technology in its review. This had the effect of diluting any positive results and damning modern incarnations of the Test by associating them with antiquated forms.

By including in their evaluation an outdated technology, the authors were able to dilute the impact of the most relevant modern tests. This was like someone reviewing

---

§§§§ Alberts followed his mentor Sydney Salmon in becoming President of the University of Arizona Cancer Center, Tucson, in his case in 2005.

the viability of hybrid automobiles by focusing on the 1980 Briggs & Stratton prototype with its eight horse-power electric motor. It would not be surprising if such a review came up with less than enthusiastic conclusions.

Despite this fact, even the reviewers found in the aggregate that "8 of the 12 articles they evaluated revealed positive results for assay-directed chemotherapy vs. empiric selection; one revealed negative results; two reveal comparable results, and one lacked a comparator arm."[276] Thus, even this unfair and inflexible evaluation revealed predominately positive effects. The reviewers rejected such positive findings out of hand.

Overall, this rejection by ASCO (the collective voice of America's 30,000 oncologists) had a devastating effect on the field of the Test. It is primarily this evaluation that most oncologists are referring to when they tell patients, "Save your money, we evaluated the Test years ago and it didn't work."

Oddly, the 2004 review claimed to have confirmed the earlier findings of a peer-reviewed article in ASCO's *Journal of Clinical Oncology* five years earlier.[277] "The Working Group's review of the literature found that little has changed since the review published by Cortazar and Johnson in 1999," they wrote. But actually, they *reversed the verdict* of Drs. Patricia Cortazar and Bruce E. Johnson's peer-reviewed discussion, for that review had concluded:

"The data accumulated thus far show that *in vitro*-selected chemotherapy seems to be *at least as effective* as empiric therapy. The technologies for selecting chemotherapeutic regimens are *well established*" (emphasis added).[278]

So, if "little had changed" in the interim, why come to diametrically opposite conclusions?

There were several other major flaws in the ASCO review. The most important of these was the failure to differentiate between clonogenic assays (which focus on stopping cell growth) and apoptotic assays (which focus on inducing programmed cell death). As I have stated, this difference is the fundamental 'line in the sand' between the two major types of tests. Although it may be a cliché by now to say so,[279] the discovery of apoptosis and programmed cell death (PCD) represent a true paradigm shift in all of biology, including but not limited to the way the Test is conducted.

It is an extraordinary fact that the ASCO reviewers started their paper with a flawed definition of the meaning of the Test. Here is their definition:

"A chemotherapy sensitivity assay refers to any *in vitro* laboratory analysis that is performed specifically to evaluate *whether tumor growth is inhibited* by a known chemotherapy drug or, more commonly, a panel of drugs"[280] (emphasis added).

But, as I have already shown, this definition is outdated. Tests that detect signs of PCD including apoptosis (which have been practiced for more than two decades) emphatically do not rely on "inhibiting tumor growth." Their proponents do not believe that inhibiting tumor growth is a meaningful metric. They are interested in agents that induce programmed cell death (PCD).

But the ASCO reviewers, influenced as they apparently were by the veterans of the clonogenic era in their ranks, simply did not embrace the fundamental difference between growth inhibition (which is measured in the clonogenic and other early assays) and modern cell-death end points. Indeed, the words 'apoptosis' and 'programmed cell death' do not even occur in this eight-page paper.

Cell death, as Nagourney pointed out, "serves as an *in vitro* surrogate for drug-induced apoptosis, the most relevant of biologic measures, and must not be confused with older growth-based end points."[281] Not surprisingly, most of their subsequent errors flowed from this fundamental mistake in defining the nature of the Test.

A New Criterion

In the 2004 ASCO review, the authors, perhaps for the first time in medical history, demanded that a laboratory test be not only sensitive and specific but also that advocates prove beyond a reasonable doubt that it extends patients' lives compared to standard 'empiric' chemotherapy. This novel requirement raised the bar higher than what other laboratory tests had ever had to prove.

It was, to quote Nagourney, "a new criterion that has never been applied previously to clinical tests."[282] As I have shown, the test for the estrogen receptor (ER), which is universally used in helping to determine treatment for breast cancer, never had to meet this exacting a standard before being adopted and approved. Neither did the CT or PET scan nor the familiar Kirby-Bauer method of screening for effective antibacterial drugs have to clear such a hurdle. In all such cases, these tests "would be hard pressed to meet this parochial definition of utility" (Nagourney).[283]

The ASCO panel also criticized the Test from a number of other directions. Some of the criticisms were patently outdated at the time they were issued, while others were merely bizarre.

Low Evaluability Rate?

The ASCO panel claimed that the Test as a rule cannot be used to evaluate an adequate percentage of samples that are submitted for testing. This was indeed, as we have seen, one of the persistent problems with the clonogenic assay, and some of the other older tests. Again, perhaps it was the inclusion of experts on the defunct clonogenic assay, and the concomitant exclusion of all practitioners of PCD-based modern tests, that led to this odd conclusion.

Poor evaluability is simply no longer characteristic of modern PCD-based tests, where the great preponderance of viable specimens are routinely and successfully analyzed in a week or so. Nagourney reports that of the thousands of specimens processed by his laboratory, "90 percent are assessable for an average of 12 to 16 drugs or combinations."[284] Similarly, in their 2008 study in the journal *Breast,* Kim *et al.* of Seoul, reported a 93 percent success rate in carrying out their form of the Test. [285]

Some of the ASCO reviewers seemed to be projecting their own frustrations with the bygone era of clonogenic testing onto the modern tests. But this charge of low evaluability is not just incorrect but bizarre to anyone who has had day-to-day experience with modern chemosensitivity testing laboratories.

Like members of the general public, advocates of modern versions of the Test were restricted to submitting letters to the *JCO* after substantial damage had been done by the ASCO article. Had they been included in the review process they could have cleared up these misconceptions and the outcome might have been very different indeed.

Slow Turnaround Rate?

The ASCO reviewers also referred to the *slow turnaround rate* with the Test. As can be easily ascertained, this charge is also outdated and wrong. As Roberto Angioli, MD, *et al.* wrote in a 2004 textbook on gynecological cancer, while the HTCA clonogenic assay did require three to four weeks for completion, most other tests are expeditious, "requiring 4 to 10 days to attain assay results."[286]

At Exiqon (formerly Oncotech), the testing period is 7 to 10 days. Rational Therapeutics, which employs a 72-hour assay, routinely provides their clients with written results by the seventh day following receipt of tissue,[287] while Cell Biolabs provides results in 6 to 8 days.[288] DiaTech analyzes specimens in just *48 to 72 hours.*[289]

So, as a rule, from start to finish, modern-day Testing takes about one week, which is a remarkable achievement. This is similar to the turnaround time for some long-established laboratory tests, such as estrogen receptors (ER) or prostate specific antigen (PSA). The testing period at most modern chemosensitivity testing laboratories, therefore, allows ample time for prompt decision-making by patients and physicians.

Apparently a turnaround time of almost two weeks does not rule out tests based on genomic principles, since ASCO's 2007 Clinical Guidelines on the Use of Tumor Markers in Breast Cancer approved the routine use of the genomic test Oncotype DX™.[290] Meanwhile, Genomic

Health states that its Oncotype DX test requires a turn-around of 10 to 14 days.[291]

Once again, the ASCO reviewers criticized a characteristic of the outdated Test of a bygone era. Most of those pokey assays were already no longer commercially available at the time of the ASCO evaluation. Meanwhile, the panelists ignored the rapid modern tests, which routinely get results back to consumers in a week or so.

Criticizing this aspect of the report, John Fruehauf, MD, of the University of California, Irvine, stated: "Citing discarded technologies as a rationale for dismissing more recent accomplishments of the field lacks the scientific rigor one expects from peer-reviewed literature."[292]

Loss of Novel Options?

Another claim of the ASCO reviewers was that the wide-scale use of the Test would lead to a "failure to identify novel options."[293] What exactly was the panel implying? Perhaps that if the Test became universally accepted it would obviate the need for clinical trials, and that this fact would lead to a decline in new drug development? If this was their meaning, it was bizarre.

First, no one has suggested that all clinical trials immediately cease in deference to the Test. As the late University of Pittsburgh biostatistician H. Samuel

Wieand, PhD,*****stated in a published critique of the ASCO report:

"CSRAs [chemosensitivity and resistance assays, ed.] are not proposed as an alternative to empiric therapy, but rather an enhancement to help identify the most effective treatment for an individual when multiple options exist...."[294]

As a matter of fact, some novel drug combinations had already emerged from chemosensitivity laboratories at the time the ASCO reviewers wrote. The most prominent of these was the combination of gemcitabine and cisplatin, so-called "Gem-Cis," which was identified and popularized by Robert Nagourney in the course of his form of the Test.[295,296]

Nagourney's paper on Gem-Cis, published in the *JCO* in 2000, has now been cited by 100 other authors[297] and led to an interest in this doublet in a variety of situations. It is presently the subject of 94 ongoing clinical trials.[298] So one can hardly argue that the approval of the Test *per se* would lead to some sort of crisis in identifying new drug combinations. Since the Test can be used to identify potential new agents, it could in fact lead to an *expansion* in potential treatments. The Test adds a powerful new

***

***** Wieand knew from whence he spoke. He was the deputy editor for statistics of ASCO's *Journal of Clinical Oncology (JCO)*.

weapon to the methods that scientists use to identify useful drugs and drug combinations.

As Jean Sargent, PhD, of Pembury Hospital in Kent, England, has written:

"Currently, drugs under development are initially selected by their effect on experimental tumour models....Possible candidates are further selected by more experimental modeling. If the agent appears effective in this system then the drug goes straight to the clinic to be tested in drug trials in patients. We firmly believe such novel agents should be tested in the laboratory against tumour cells taken directly from patients to complement the other tests and confirm their effectiveness before they are given to patients."[299]

This improbable charge could have been readily dispelled had they allowed input from outside experts in the field of apoptosis-based assays.

Despite the prejudiced manner in which the Test was evaluated, the TEC reviewers (who partnered with the ASCO authors in this project) admitted:

"Higher response rates were observed in most studies for assay-guided patients compared with those treated empirically, though differences were not always statistically significant."[300]

The reader should ponder these words. Despite the insurance industry origin of the TEC review, in the end even these reviewers admitted that most of the patients whose drugs were chosen by the Test had more beneficial responses than those whose treatment were guided by the standard recommendations, i.e., the empirically guided group.

But that fact alone was not sufficient to sway these reviewers of the Test. Suddenly, they decided that *all* such trials also had to be *statistically significant for survival* in order to receive a stamp of approval, or rather to avoid the *ex cathedra* rejection, of ASCO and of Blue Cross/Blue Shield's technology panel.

We should ask therefore how many other procedures or treatments in oncology have been proven of statistically significant benefit in all or even most tests? I will speak about results in the chemotherapy of lung cancer in some detail. But does the reader think that this is the case with surgery or radiation therapy?

Much of what is recommended in these time-honored medical specialties is supported by the results of retrospective case series, not RCTs. Readers who doubt this should consult the excellent 2008 textbook, *Radiation Oncology: An Evidence-Based Approach.*[301] This book is unusual in that it grades each treatment recommendation based on the strength of the scientific evidence. The reader may be surprised to see how many current treatments are not actually supported by high-grade empirical results from rigorous clinical trials. For example, radiotherapy is often recommended for the adjuvant treatment of pancreatic cancer. But this earns a grade of C, meaning that while there is some evidence from non-randomized studies, the data is inconsistent.[302]

Another example is low-dose rate brachytherapy (a kind of radiotherapy) for prostate cancer, which receives a grade of D, meaning there is "little or no systemic empirical evidence" to support the recommendation.[303]

How about chemotherapy, the mainstay of the medical oncology profession? Have *all* of its currently approved indications been proven, in statistically significant RCTs, to extend progression-free or overall survival?

Since this is the standard to which the Test is now being held, let us take a moment to review one situation that has been much in the news. On February 22, 2008, the FDA granted accelerated approval for the drug bevacizumab (Avastin®, manufactured by Genentech) in combination with paclitaxel (Taxol®), in the treatment of patients who have not received chemotherapy for metastatic HER2-negative breast cancer.

Has Avastin been proven to extend overall survival in this patient population? In late 2007, the FDA's Oncology Drug Advisory Committee (ODAC) ruled that it was not and recommended against approval for this indication.

But the FDA commissioner at the time, Andrew von Eschenbach, MD, overruled his own panel's recommendation, although the main clinical trial, performed at Indiana University, had showed that "initial therapy of metastatic breast cancer with paclitaxel plus bevacizu-mab prolongs progression-free survival, *but not overall survival,* as compared with paclitaxel alone"[304] (emphasis added).

In another clinical trial, published in the *JCO* in 2005, the addition of Avastin to the drug capecitabine added nothing in terms of improvement in either progression-free or overall survival.[305] Also, when Avastin was added to docetaxel (Taxotere®) in locally advanced breast cancer there was "no difference in overall clinical response, pro-gression-free survival, or overall survival."[306]

Yet at its 2008 annual meeting ASCO hailed the ex-panded use of Avastin at a press conference because, in one study, compared with a docetaxel alone, Avastin somewhat improved progression-free survival, which is not the same as the more meaningful parameter, overall survival.[307]

So, far from showing a statistically significant survival benefit, the trials to date do not support Avastin's ability to actually increase overall survival in breast cancer (at least when administered in empiric fashion). Yet Avastin's global sales totaled $6 billion in 2009 and Genentech is a major contributor to ASCO and its annual meeting.[308] In one year alone the data from over 200 ab-stracts in 20 types of cancer were presented on Genen-tech's oncology products, "demonstrating our leadership in the field," said the company.[309]

I would suggest that there is a double standard at work when advocates of a blockbuster drug, such as Avastin, are able to get ASCO's enthusiastic endorsement, despite an almost total absence of evidence that it extends overall survival. (FDA simultaneously lowered the threshold for approval of other cancer drugs, according to the *New York Times*.[310])

Meanwhile, advocates of the Test, a laboratory procedure, are told they have to demonstrate through *unanimously* positive clinical trials that they can *extend overall survival* in each and every case. They must do this to the satisfaction of reviewers who have no personal experience with the modern tests that are in common use, and despite the fact that advocates of PCD-based tests were systematically excluded from participating in the evaluation process.[311]

There was thus a glaring discrepancy between the way other approved tests were treated and the unreasonable demands suddenly made of the Test. This violates the long-standing principle of "equal justice under the law," a principle so central that it is etched above the entrance to the US Supreme Court.[312]

This was not always the case. On previous occasions, Medicare reviewers had actively sought and considered commentaries and testimony from experts on modern era testing (see below). But in the 2004 ASCO review, there was neither open debate between proponents and opponents, nor the chance for transparent discussions or public input. To those who watched from the sidelines this gave a strong impression that the condemnation of the Test was a foregone conclusion.

Cost of RCTs vs. the Test

"One major issue that is the proverbial 'elephant in the room' is the enormous regulatory burden associated with opening and running clinical trials and the resulting cost required to manage this burden," wrote George Weiner, MD, of the University of Iowa cancer center in 2009.[313]

In 2006, it was estimated that to enroll a single patient in a phase III trial cost the sponsor $26,000.[314] An adequately powered RCT might need 1,000 patients. (See discussion of NSCLC, below.) So the cost of such a trial would be around $26 million. NCI (with its over $5.15 billion funding in FY 2010[315]) has the money but has never deigned to fund a randomized trial of the Test.†††††

Think of that the next time someone glibly demands randomized controlled trials to prove the value of the Test. Someone has to pay for those proposed trials, but

††††† NCI's annual operating budget in FY 2008 was $4.83 billion. Its operating budget in FY 2009 was $4.96 billion. But the American Recovery and Investment Act of 2009 provided NCI with an additional $1.267 billion to spend.

those who most vociferously demand them have so far never volunteered to do so.

Why don't the laboratories that perform the Test themselves fund the trials? The simple answer is that they do not have either the resources or the economic motivation. That is because most of the technology involved in the practice of the Test is in the public domain. According to Weisenthal:

"It must be understood that none of the above technologies are truly proprietary, in the sense that existing patents are not defensible, in my opinion, and that, in any event, there are workaround solutions available to anyone who wants to perform assays based on the above principles."[316]

Thus no one can reap an adequate reward for his or her efforts should the testing turn out positive. DiaTech Labs has sponsored a few small, non-randomized trials. But they have licensed a proprietary form of the Test from Vanderbilt University and therefore hope to profit from its wide-scale adoption.

But, generally speaking, the person who pays for the clinical trial will probably not be able to profit directly from the results, because of their inability to secure a legal monopoly on the technology through the patent process. It is the same issue that bedevils proposed trials of various inexpensive and generically available natural therapies. (I refer interested readers to my book, *The Cancer Industry*.[317])

Role of Insurance Industry

I have mentioned that the ASCO review considered only a total of 12 papers and that all favorable correlative studies were excluded from the start as a matter of principle.

John Fruehauf, MD, of the University of California Irvine Cancer Center pointed out in a letter to the *JCO* that the origin of the ASCO review process was a previous article sponsored by the Aetna Life and Casualty Company.[318] But Aetna, Blue Cross/Blue Shield and other health insurance companies have a vested interest in the outcome of such a study, i.e., they have an economic motive to favor a negative outcome. This is because they are notorious at balking to pay for new tests. Fruehauf comments:

"An informed reader wonders how an industry-sponsored selection of 12 papers could be considered an adequate representation of a literature composed of some 790 peer-reviewed articles (according to PubMed search on 'chemosensitivity assays'). It should be noted that some members of the American Society of Clinical Oncology (ASCO) panel withdrew from authorship on the basis of their view that the panel's conclusions were not balanced. The majority of citations offered are significantly flawed and of only historical interest."[319]

Yet this is the flawed ASCO review that essentially damned the Test from the time it was published until the present day.

The insurance industry has not always been entirely unreceptive to the Test. In the past, some industry leaders have grasped the value of such testing and have tried to offer it for their members. In the 1990s, it was common for such private insurance companies as Prudential, Principal Mutual, State Farm, Connecticut General, etc., to pay fully for these tests.[320] Other companies paid for at least part of the expense.

In October 1993 and March 1994 the issue of reimbursement was vigorously debated at meetings of the Blue Shield of California Medical Policy Committee on Quality and Technology, held in San Francisco. In the debate of March 2, 1994, an odd situation developed as representatives of the *Southern* California Oncology Association (some of whose members used the Test) came out in strong support of reimbursement while the *Northern* California Oncology Association initially opposed reimbursement and claimed that the Test was merely investigational. After vigorous debate, however, the final vote was 20 to 0 in favor of reimbursement. It was an impressive display of the fact that when the proponents of PCD-based testing could meet their opponents in open debate, they could prevail.

In fact, the official Blue Shield of California conclusion was as follows: "Drug resistance testing in oncology is accurate and reliable. This information can affect clinical decision-making and can lead to the avoidance of ineffective and potentially harmful chemotherapeutic agents. Although there are few prospective clinical trials comparing standard therapy with chemotherapy chosen by *in vitro* assay, there are sufficient published data to determine their safety, clinical utility, and impact on clinical decision making. Recommendation: It is recommended that the human tumor drug resistance assay is eligible for coverage when this information is required for the selection of chemotherapy."[321]

However, this recommendation was not to stand. Essentially, it fell victim to the ASCO and Blue Cross TEC reviews of 2004, which after that point were universally used to justify denial of reimbursement for the Test.

It was ill omened that ASCO chose to base this influential report on a medical industry-sponsored selection of 12 papers. The role of the insurance industry in the 2004 'ASCO fiasco' needs to be examined. There are many instances in which the insurance industry has pursued a short-term strategy of denying the need for valid procedures, on both an individual and societal level. Much of this information emerged in the course of the national debate over health policy that dominated the political dialogue for much of 2009 and 2010, leading up to passage of the Patient Protection and Affordable Care Act.

For instance, in June 2009 executives of three of the nation's largest health insurers told federal lawmakers that they would continue canceling medical coverage for some sick policyholders, "despite withering criticism from Republican and Democratic members of Congress who decried the practice as unfair and abusive."[322] Their policy, known as rescission, "has left thousands of Americans burdened with costly medical bills despite paying insurance premiums," according to the *Los Angeles Times*.[323]

Congressional investigators found (the *Los Angeles Times* continued):

"Policyholders with breast cancer, lymphoma and more than 1,000 other conditions were targeted for rescission and that employees were praised in performance reviews for terminating the policies of customers with expensive illnesses."[324]

Many other abuses by the health insurance industry could be cited, and most have this in common: they sacrifice the greater good—of sick patients, of society, even of their own long-term interests—for the immediate goal of making profits (often by ruthlessly cutting costs) in the short-term. I believe that the rejection of the Test has the same roots, the rejection of the long-term interests of cancer patients (and of the industry itself) for the sake of shortsighted goals.

VI. WHAT'S WRONG WITH CHEMO?

If the current conventional way of delivering anticancer drugs were very successful one might be inclined to leave well enough alone, and not tinker in fundamental ways with how drugs are chosen for treatment. One doesn't hear too many demands these days for alternatives to the polio vaccine.

However, as I shall demonstrate, there is something fundamentally wrong with the way that chemotherapy is chosen for most patients. In most clinics and hospitals, patients with a specific diagnosis and stage of illness are generally given the same basic chemotherapy regimen. With some inevitable adjustments for body size, age, sex, and a few other factors, all patients are then treated in "cookbook" fashion.

The cookbook in question may vary, of course, as oncologists can chose from regimens suggested by various authoritative sources, such as the National Comprehensive Cancer Network (NCCN), the American Society of Clinical Oncology (ASCO), the NCI Web site (www.cancer.gov), or perhaps their favorite textbook. With around 30,000 oncologists, there is naturally some variation from center to center, state to state, and country to country, but in almost all cases the doctors follow one cookbook or another. Those who don't may chose drugs based on even worse criteria—including the "chemotherapy concession," discussed below.

But after 40 years of the official US government War on Cancer, progress in successfully combating the statistically major forms of cancer, including the common solid tumors of adults, has been agonizingly slow. The death rates for most advanced cancer remain high and, according to some observers, are approximately the same as they were when the War on Cancer began in December 1971.[325,326]

One could write a book about the limitations of chemotherapy in the treatment of common cancers. In fact, 15 years ago I published such a book, *Questioning Chemotherapy*.[327] The situation has not changed substantially in the past decade and a half. I will illustrate the gravity of the problem by considering in some detail the chemotherapeutic treatment of America's most frequently fatal form of malignancy.

The Case of NSCLC

We have already seen what the Test can achieve in the case of both non-small cell and small cell lung cancer (see above). I now want to illustrate the current impasse in selecting drugs in empiric fashion by considering the treatment of non-small cell lung cancer (NSCLC), America's most deadly cancer.

According to the American Cancer Society (ACS), in the US in 2010 there were 222,520 new cases of carcinoma of the lung or bronchus and 157,300 deaths.[328]

The major and preventable cause is tobacco smoking. Under the microscope, 85 percent of these tumors were classified as having non-small cell histology. Although lung cancers caught early may be cured through multi-modal therapy, this is rarely the case with late-stage disease. Since 40 percent of NSCLC patients present with stage IV (metastasized) disease, about 100,000 Americans per year have an advanced and presumably incurable form of this illness.

After decades of researching and utilizing chemotherapy, the survival rate in late-stage NSCLC remains poor. There are, however, some drugs that are active against the disease. A few decades ago, scientists noted that drugs that incorporate the mineral platinum sometimes had an anti-cancer effect in this type of cancer.

It was later noted that taxanes (drugs derived from the Pacific yew tree), as well as some other agents, such as gemcitabine (Gemzar), also had a beneficial effect against some patients' tumors.

According to the NCI, randomized controlled trials (RCTs) "have shown that cisplatin-based chemotherapy improves survival and palliates disease-related symptoms."[329] The administration of a platinum-based drug also generally includes another drug, such as a taxane or gemcitabine, in what is called a "doublet." In addition, NCI says, patients who have certain favorable characteristics‡‡‡‡ may also benefit from the addition of the targeted anti-angiogenic drug bevacizumab (Avastin) to the doublet.

So far, these recommendations seem straightforward. But how effective is this form of chemotherapy? When NCI states that a drug "improves survival and palliates disease-related symptoms," what exactly does it mean? And does this apply to everybody, or only to a select minority? We can get some idea by looking at a 2009 randomized controlled trial published in ASCO's *Journal of Clinical Oncology.*

The authors, European thoracic oncologists, set out to see if various doses of Avastin (bevacizumab) improved survival when added to the doublet of carboplatin and gemcitabine, a combination known as CG + Avastin. All patients received six cycles of CG and were then randomized to receive (a) low-dose Avastin, (b) high-dose Avastin, or an inert placebo every three weeks until the cancer progressed. Over a thousand patients were enrolled in this trial, so it was sufficiently 'powered' to detect even small differences in survival.

What was the objective response rate (which the World Health Organization defines as a shrinkage of tumor by

---

‡‡‡‡ These favorable factors are a non-squamous histology, good performance status, no history of coughing up blood or other bleeding, and no recent history of cardiovascular events.

50 percent or more for one month or more)? It was 20.1 percent in the CG + placebo group, 34.1 percent in the low-dose Avastin plus CG group and 30.4 percent in the high-dose Avastin plus CG group.

Meanwhile, median progression free survival (PFS) was *6.1 months* for the group that received CG plus placebo vs. *6.5 months* in those who received either low-dose or high-dose Avastin. Thus, the benefit of adding Avastin in this study was 0.4 months of progression free survival (PFS). Because of the size of the trial, this absolute benefit of *12-day* improvement in PFS was "statistically significant."§§§§§,330

Avastin at either dose *did* help shrink more tumors, but (as often happens) there was little correlation between the response rate and improvement in progression-free survival (see Table 8).

Table 8
CG With or Without Avastin in NSCLC:
Results of a Randomized Trial

	Response Rate (%)	PFS Duration
CG + placebo	20.1	6.1 mos.
CG + low-dose Avastin	34.1	6.5 mos.
CG + high-dose Avastin	30.4	6.5 mos.

CG = cisplatin + gemcitabine; PFS = progression-free survival.
Data from: *J Clin Oncol.* 2009;27:1227-1234.

---

§§§§§ No data was yet available on overall survival, but it is unlikely to be much more positive than for progression-free survival.

Oncologists tend to be sanguine when it comes to inter-preting the results of their own clinical trials. These European authors were no exception, claiming that Avastin "significantly improved" PFS and the objective response rate and that Avastin plus platinum-based che-motherapy "offers clinical benefit for bevacizumab-eligible patients with advanced NSCLC."[331] One wonders how "significant" this clinical benefit of *12-day improvement* in PFS was for the patients themselves, especially since it also involved considerable toxicity.

The Vanderbilt Trial: Another RCT, performed in 2006 at Vanderbilt University, Nashville, administered the doublet of carboplatin + taxol (CT) vs. CT + Avastin. This too was a relatively large study, with 878 patients with advanced (stage IIIB or IV) NSCLC.[332] In this trial, the median overall survival was 10.3 months in the chemo-therapy-alone group vs. 12.3 months in the Avastin-added group. Thus there was a two-month overall survival (OS) benefit to Avastin.

The median progression-free survival (PFS) in the two groups was 4.5 months for chemotherapy-alone vs. 6.2 months in the Avastin-added group. Thus there was a 1.7-month improvement achieved with the addition of Avastin. This was similar to the 6.5 months progression-free survival seen in the European study of CG + Avastin, above. However, the adverse effects were also more fre-quent and in fact there were 15 treatment-related deaths in the Avastin-added group, including five from pulmonary hemorrhages.[333]

I want to make two points about these studies (which are representative of a number of similar trials):

First, despite 40 years of trying, *empirically determined* chemotherapy regimens still do not work very well for advanced NSCLC. A median progression-free survival of six months, or an overall survival of twelve months, is a disappointing outcome. In fact, it is hard to believe this is the best the medical profession can do for more than 100,000 people diagnosed with advanced-stage NSCLC every year (in the US alone). Whether its practitioners acknowledge it or not, oncology is in desperate need of better treatment approaches.

Second, only a minority of non-small cell lung cancer patients responds to chemotherapeutic regimens that are chosen on the basis of RCTs. In the 2009 European trial discussed above only 34.1 percent of patients responded to the various combinations, while in the Vanderbilt trial a similar 35 percent responded.[334] Put another way, *about two-thirds of patients do not respond at all.* Standard chemotherapy was therefore given to these individuals in vain.

When NCI says that "cisplatin-based chemotherapy improves survival and palliates disease-related symptoms,[335] it is referring to the results achieved on average in one-third of patients. The rest are not helped, in fact they are potentially harmed, by taking this 'average' therapy.

I could easily extend this discussion to the treatment of advanced cancers of the liver, pancreas and gall bladder, kidney, esophagus, stomach, brain, etc. Lest you think that I have stacked the deck by focusing on one particularly difficult-to-treat cancer, consider the words of two leading oncologists. Writing in the famous DeVita textbook, they stated: "Although 30 percent of patients with solid tumors respond to aggressive combination chemotherapy...the vast majority are resistant."[336],******

There are of course bright spots and exceptions to the rule. But what I have outlined for NSCLC is a fairly typical response rate in patients with advanced epithelial cancers.

My point is not to 'bash' chemotherapy but to ask: Could one convert many of these non-responders into responders? This is the great promise of the Test. Had a portion of these same patients' cancer cells been removed through surgery or biopsy, and then studied outside their bodies *(ex vivo)* in advance of treatment, then two beneficial things could have happened:

****** Although these words were written in 1999, I believe they are equally valid today.

Those whose cells were shown to be resistant to particular drugs could have been identified and those ineffective drug could have been avoided;

Those whose cells were sensitive to particular drugs could have been identified and they could have been given only the drugs that had the greatest chance of success.

Judging by a large amount of past experience, this would have raised the number of responders well above one-third. Meanwhile, those whose cells exhibited extreme drug resistance, and did not respond to any drugs, could have been spared unnecessary toxic treatment, which killed 15 patients in the Vanderbilt clinical trial (above). They would be good candidates for more experimental treatments.

Again, I urge the reader to reconsider the results achieved using the Test in both non-small cell and small cell lung cancer. I think the potential of this approach becomes apparent when one contrasts that to the results using empiric therapy.

Off Label Use

At the present time, many doctors are seeking ways of escaping the constraints of one-size-fits all empiric therapy. The trouble is that many of them are casting around in an irrational manner, using drugs that have no intrinsic connection to their patient's actual tumors. This raises the widespread problem of off-label use. According to writer Merrill Goozner:

"Many of the nation's 30,000 oncologists are engaged in what could be described as an unobserved and uncontrolled science experiment, especially when it comes to treating the 560,000 Americans who die each year from the more than 100 forms of the disease. As these patients' cancers advance, their physicians try regimens they read about in journals or hear about from colleagues. The outcomes are never gathered. The data is never analyzed. And the findings are never disseminated."[337]

Oftentimes, a cancer diagnosis presents both physicians and patients with therapeutic choices that are agonizing in their uncertainty. Even the so-called curable malignancies, such as acute forms of leukemia and lymphoma, are treated with various combinations, each of which emphasizes specific classes of drugs, but sometimes without clear-cut guidance as to which drugs in each category are best.

Each of the approved chemotherapeutic drugs has its approved indications but at the same time the FDA makes no effort to stop doctors from using these same drugs in an "off label" way. In other words, every new drug is available for doctors to use on *all* of their cancer patients. According to Goozner, about 70 percent of all cancer drugs are administered in this off-label fashion, unsupervised by the FDA. "Much of the off-label use is supported by the slimmest of evidence," Goozner says, "often just a single trial in the medical literature of limited size and duration."[338]

"Most of off-label use is done with good intentions," adds University of Chicago oncologist Richard Schilsky, MD, the 2009 president of the American Society of Clinical Oncology (ASCO). But, he adds, "no data is collected on whether it's an effective strategy or not. And most of it gets reimbursed."[339] Thus the manner in which cancer drugs are chosen tends to be anarchic.

William McGuire thought the abundance of drugs disturbing in 1994 when, he wrote, with evident exasperation, that *one or two* new antineoplastic agents were being introduced *every other year*. Imagine the situation today as the number of FDA approved drugs has proliferated. In recent years, in fact, the FDA has been granting about *a dozen* new drug approvals to treat cancer each and every year!

Here, from the FDA's Web site, is a list of the drugs that the agency has approved in recent years:

Recently FDA Approved Anticancer Agents
Anastrozole (Arimidex®)
Azacitidine (Vidaza®)
Bevacizumab (Avastin™)
Bicalutamide (Casodex®)
Bortezomib (Velcade®)

Capecitabine (Xeloda®)

Carboplatin (Paraplatin®)

Cetuximab (Erbitux™)

Dasatinib (Sprycel™)

Docetaxel (Taxotere®)

Doxorubicin Liposomal (Doxil®Caelyx®)

Epirubicin (Ellence®)

Erlotinib (Tarceva®)

Exemestane (Aromasin®)

Gefitinib (Iressa®)

Gemcitabine (Gemzar®)

Goserelin (Zoladex®)

Imatinib, STI-571 (Gleevec®)

Irinotecan (Camptosar®)

Lapatinib (Tykerb)

Letrozole (Femara®)

Oxaliplatin (Eloxatin™)

Paclitaxel (Onxol™Paxene®Taxol®)

Pemetrexed (Alimta®)

Rituximab (Rituxan®)

Sorafenib (Nexavar®)

Sunitinib (Sutent®)

Tamoxifen (Nolvadex ®)

Temozolomide (Temodar®)

Trastuzumab (Herceptin®)

Triptorelin (Trelstar™ Depot)

Navelbine®

Data from FDA web site

In addition to the newer agents there are many older drugs that were approved decades ago but that are still in common use, such as the cyclophosphamide (Cytoxan), 5-fluorouracil (5-FU or Efudex), doxorubicin (Adriamycin) and methotrexate (Trexall). Oftentimes various agents are administered in two, three or four drug combinations, in what is called polychemotherapy.

This creates a welter of effects and adverse (side) effects, whose net result in any particular patient is impossible to decipher.

Obviously, the possibilities are endless. How is an oncologist supposed to choose meaningfully among so many different agents, without the use of a test that predicts what will work, or fail to work, in any particular patient? This is the nightmarish predicament of oncologists who try to divine which combination of drugs is likely to be most beneficial and least toxic for any particular patient. No wonder they fall back on the recommendations of authorities, such as the NCCN.

But this one-treatment-fits-all philosophy (by which the same drugs are chosen for all patients with a particular diagnosis) is a violation of the fundamental rule of "biochemical individuality," which was elucidated by Roger J. Williams, PhD, half a century ago.[340]

Ideally, an oncologist needs to take into account each individual's unique characteristics, down to the molecular level. First and foremost, that means assaying the sensitivity of the patient's tumor to the drugs in question through the Test. Trying to understand an individual's likely response to treatment without predictive laboratory tests is like the ancient mariner who tried to navigate the "Ocean Sea" without sextant or compass.

Meta-Analyses

Since the results of clinical trials can and do differ one from another, statisticians sometimes perform *meta-analyses* in an attempt to reconcile disparate results. Meta-analyses are not trials in themselves, but combine the results of various clinical trials in order to summarize disparate findings and extract usable conclusions from a welter of information.

At one time meta-analyses were seen as a virtual panacea that would solve the problem of conflicting clinical trials.[341] But, alas, meta-analyses also can and do differ in their conclusions, requiring yet further analyses of meta-analyses! "In theory, aggregation of data from multiple trials should enhance the precision and accuracy of any pooled result," the *British Medical Journal* editorialized in 1997. "But combining data requires a leap of faith: it presumes that the differences among studies are primarily due to chance. In fact, differences in the direction or size of treatment effects may be caused by other factors."[342]

In other words, clinical trials can differ greatly in their intrinsic quality, and combining good and bad trials may only confound the issue. Often, this convoluted, expensive and time-consuming process of meta-analysis only leads to greater confusion.

To take a single instance, again in the case of NSCLC, the NCI's attempt to summarize the current state of knowledge is valiant but ultimately sows confusion. At its Web site, www.cancer.gov, NCI reviewers attempt to reconcile the result of three separate meta-analyses, each of which had evaluated nine or ten clinical trials.

Some of trials were published studies, but others never saw the light of day but for the sake of completeness in the meta-analysis were retrieved from file drawers where they reposed for months or years. The NCI then had to compare these various trials, as well as these meta-analyses, in regards to responses, overall survival, progression-free survival, and the toxicity of regimens containing two, three or more drugs.

Remember that each meta-analysis itself wrestled with the results of trials in which hundreds of patients took part, patients who often had quite different personal characteristics, not to mention the inherent heterogeneity of tumors, even in the same diagnostic category.

This effort has lead to the modern-day equivalent of determining how many angels can dance on the head of a pin. But even the great St. Thomas Aquinas might have thrown up his hands in frustration if he had to reconcile such disparate and contradictory results. For mere mortals of the 21st century it is an impossible task.

After delving into the minutiae of the various meta-analyses, the NCI finally reaches the following conclusions about empiric treatment results in NSCLC:

1. Platinum combinations with vinorelbine, paclitaxel, docetaxel, gemcitabine, irinotecan, and pemetrexed yield similar improvements in survival. Types and frequencies of toxic effects differ, and these may determine the preferred regimen for an individual patient.

2. Cisplatin and carboplatin yield similar improvements in outcome, although some (but not all) trials and meta-analyses of trials suggest that outcomes with cisplatin may be superior, although with a higher risk of certain toxicities such as nausea and vomiting.

3. Non-platinum combinations offer no advantage to platinum-based chemotherapy, and some studies demonstrate inferiority.

4. Three-drug combinations of the commonly used chemotherapy drugs do not result in superior survival and are more toxic than two-drug combinations.

5. Certain three-drug combinations that add so-called targeted agents may result in superior survival.

Imagine being an oncologist trying to extract clear-cut treatment recommendations from such guidelines. The NCI write-up also delicately sidesteps the unacknowledged fact that these "improvements in survival" are generally measured in weeks. There is also no real guidance here on how the "types and frequency" of toxic effects from various drug combinations can possibly guide treatment.

At the end of the day, here is NCI's takeaway message:

"Among the active combinations, definitive recommendations regarding drug dose and schedule cannot be made.... *No specific regimen can be regarded as standard therapy"* (emphasis added).

So here, at the end of a truly massive intellectual effort, NCI's experts conclude...that they cannot reach a conclusion about the dose or schedule.

This comes more than 30 years after the first report on the benefit of platinum-containing drugs in treating NSCLC appeared in *Cancer Treatment Reports*. NCI still cannot offer a standard regimen for this all-too-common form of cancer.[343]

If, however, we accept the recommendation of some platinum-containing drug as fundamental (and, because of its potential toxicity, not everyone does), then we have to consider that there are three platinum drugs that have been approved by the FDA: cisplatin, carboplatin and oxaliplatin (which is mainly used for colorectal cancer).

So, following the NCI's recommendation, there would still be many possible two-drug regimens (e.g., cisplatin +

vinorelbine, cisplatin + paclitaxel, cisplatin + docetaxel, etc.) potentially available for such patients (Table 9, see next page):

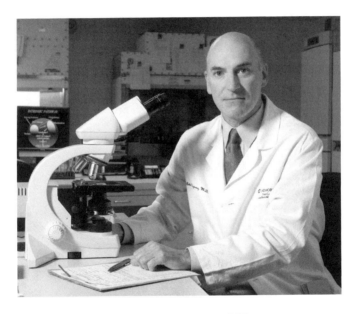

Robert A. Nagourney, MD,
founder of Rational Therapeutics, at microscope.

Table 9
PubMed-listed Articles on Platinum-containing
Combinations for NSCLC

	VIN	PAC	DOC	GEM	IRI	PMX	TOTAL
CDDP	771	685	486	819	235	84	3080
CBCDA	264	801	292	409	104	48	1918
OX	16	15	12	30	11	13	97
TOTAL	1051	1501	790	1258	350	145	5095

Data from PubMed, as of December 2009.
CBCDA = carboplatin, CDDP = cisplatin, DOC = docletaxel,
GEM = gemcitabine, IRI = irinotecan, OX = oxaliplatin,
PAC = pacletaxel, PMX = pemetrexed, PRM = pemetrexed,
VIN= vinorelbine.

According to this table, the number of PubMed-listed articles on these combinations is over 5,000. Hypothetically, if you took 15 minutes to read each of these articles, you would need to devote 150 eight-hour workdays to the process. And while you were engaged in that process, another 600 or so new articles would have appeared on the topic!

This is daunting, especially when you consider that you are now approaching the median survival time for patients with advanced NSCLC, and you have not even begun to finish reading the relevant literature, much less deciding on a treatment protocol.

But, alas, you would still not be done trying to figure out the possibilities. For NCI raises the prospect of adding other drugs, such as one or more of the anti-angiogenic or "targeted" agents to the above two-drug combinations.

There are many potential third drugs. The most commonly mentioned is Avastin (bevacizumab). But why stop there? There are numerous other third drug possibilities, such as Gleevec (imatinib mesylate), Tarceva (erlotinib), Velcade (bortezomib), Herceptin (trastuzumab), Erbitux (cetuxumab), etc. (see above list of FDA approved agents).

And the "nibs, mibs and mabs"[344] keep coming. In late 2008 it was reliably estimated that there were 373 such "molecular targeted therapies" (MTTs) in the pharmaceutical pipeline, of which 38 were in late-stage development.[345] The number of drugs increases constantly, and so too the bewildering array of therapeutic possibilities.

Even if one conservatively limits oneself to the results of published RCTs, one still comes up with a very large number of possibilities for the treatment of NSCLC, all of which have similar plausibility and results.

And this problem is not getting any better. As the number of available drugs expands, the glut of information on possible drug combinations becomes dizzying. In 1972, the first full year of the War on Cancer, there were just 167 papers on clinical trials relating to cancer, of which 26 were randomized controlled trials. In the year 2009 there were 5,208 such articles, of which 1,672 were RCTs, a manifold difference!

Information is exploding all around us. In cancer, the more than $100 billion dollars poured into cancer research since 1950 has certainly increased the amount of *information* exponentially. But has it resulted in an equivalent increase in the *knowledge* of how best to treat this very common yet very deadly form of cancer? I don't think so.

"The system is overloaded with drugs and under-loaded with wisdom and expertise for using them," David S. Alberts, MD, president of the University of Arizona Cancer Center told *Scientific American* in the course of a feature story on the Test.[346] In this explosion of information, without guidance from the Test, it actually becomes increasingly difficult for oncologists to give clear-cut advice on what treatment is likely to be most effective or the least damaging. That is the situation in which NCI, and many others, find themselves: *"Definitive recommendations…cannot be made."*

Oncologists urgently need ways of cutting through information overload and of analyzing this superfluity of data to find meaningful patterns that can guide treatment decisions.

To summarize, reliance on clinical trials for making treatment decisions has not resulted in the adoption of effective standard regimens. Rather, there is a welter of confusing recommendations over which agents to use for any particular condition. This should hardly be surprising, since every individual's tumor is unique and responds, at different points in its development, to different agents. The clinical trialist's answer to this impasse, not surprisingly, is to conduct yet more clinical trials! But further trials often result in *increased confusion* as yet more regimens are introduced as potential treatments. The Test offers a rational way out of this confusion

Rise of the Clinical Trials Industry

I believe that some of the resistance to the idea of the Test comes about because it represents a threat to another powerful segment of the medical-industrial complex. This is the burgeoning clinical trials industry. Clinical trials and the Test compete in trying to provide answers to the question of which of two or more regimens is the best for any particular patient.

The reliance on RCTs to arrive at treatment decisions has resulted in the growth of a lucrative industry. One rarely hears the conducting of trials described in economic terms, and it is difficult to arrive at firm figures for the size and scope of this industry.

Nonetheless, we get some idea from the fact that US pharmaceutical and biotechnology companies spent a total of $59 billion on research and development (R&D) in 2007.[347] As one 2010 report put it: "The recruitment of patients for clinical trials is an essential part of the complex and inherently risky R&D process for pharmaceuticals."[348]

Many of today's clinical trials are carried out by contract research organizations (CROs), which perform clinical trials in various countries on behalf of drug companies. These companies took in approximately $15 billion in 2007.[349] Oncology is their strongest area of growth, and is expected to increase by an impressive 21 percent over the next few years.[350]

Simply put, performing clinical trials to service the pharmaceutical industry has become a big and powerful business, accounting for a significant portion of the income of many individuals, including some top oncologists.

Quintiles (a leading CRO) boasts that it has 23,000 employees in more than 50 countries who have "helped develop or commercialize all of the top 30 best-selling drugs."[351] In doing so, they have enrolled more than 35,000 patients into cancer drug trials since 2004.[352]

According to www.clinicaltrials.gov, there are 31,000 active clinical trials currently recruiting patients, of which about 10,000 involve cancer.[††††††] This activity extends into every major cancer center, and many private practices, around the world.

One of the revolutionary aspects of the Test is that its wide-scale adoption would curtail the need for many of

---

[††††††] All figures are rounded off to the nearest thousand.

these RCTs. As I have tried to show, multiple options exist in the chemotherapeutic treatment of most people's cancer. It is rare for there *not* to be a dispute over the proper treatment of any type of cancer. I have shown this to be the case with NSCLC, but lung cancer is hardly unique.

For instance, a cancer whose treatment is relatively clear-cut, invasive breast cancer, also offers almost endless treatment possibilities. The NCI Web site, www.cancer.gov, contains a discussion of breast cancer drug choices that alone runs to 18 manuscript pages (4,486 words)![353]

There is no telling exactly how the Test would affect the clinical trial industry and some feel the two approaches are compatible. I have quoted above the late Prof. Wieand of Pittsburgh, who was an advocate of the Test, may have been trying to soften its revolutionary aspect, when he wrote that it was "not proposed as an alternative to empiric therapy, but rather an enhancement to help identify the most effective treatment for an individual when multiple options exist...."[354]

Since multiple therapeutic options usually exist, I see no reason why, over time, the Test would not reduce the need for many trials whose sole purpose is to compare one regimen with another. The Test *is truly a paradigm changing technology*. It also has the potential to make all of oncology more rational, cost effective and efficacious.

This would a salutary development for health care in generally, but a serious blow to the clinical trial industry, which is already in trouble because of consumer (and private physician) resistance to clinical experiments. At the present time, only between 1.3 and 1.8 percent of cancer patients enter clinical trials sponsored by the National Cancer Institute.[355]

"Participation in clinical trials remains low and is a central issue in oncology," according to a 2005 review.[356] Around the world, in Canada,[357] France,[358] the United Kingdom,[359] South Asia,[360] and the United States[361] clinical trialists bewail their inability to recruit a sufficient number of qualified patients to complete trials. In a survey of 114 UK trials, for instance, "less than one-third recruited their original target within the time originally specified...."[362] Many trials languish for years and eventually expire for lack of suitable recruits.

Oncologists bewail the wide-scale patient (and doctor) resistance to clinical trials. However, the treatment under study, and the information derived from the trial, is rarely of any practical use to individual patients, including those who enroll in the trial. In effect, such individuals are asked to altruistically offer up their ailing bodies for the good of science—and for the benefit of future generations of patients.

"Altruism and trust lie at the heart of research on human subjects," according to a 2005 statement from the

International Committee of Medical Journal Editors. "Altruistic individuals volunteer for research because they trust that their participation will contribute to improved health for others...."[363]

But if it becomes widely accepted that the Test can usually identify the optimal treatment regimen *ex vivo*, then what will happen to the already inadequate recruitment of patients for clinical trials? After all, what patient would agree to enter a clinical trial comparing two regimens, one of which has unknown value, when the answer to the question of what works best could be available for that individual within a week or so of submitting a live tumor specimen?

No one in the clinical trial business to my knowledge has come out and said that they oppose the Test because it undermines their industry. However, it is an inescapable conclusion that the Test has greater intrinsic appeal that an approach that, because of a lack of willing participants, is already on shaky ground.

The Chemotherapy Concession

There is another method of arriving at treatment decisions, other than either the Test or empiric trials. This is choosing treatment based on the personal preferences of the oncologist. This is more common than many readers are likely to realize, because of what the *New York Times* and others have called the "Chemotherapy Concession."

The Chemotherapy Concession refers to the wide-scale practice whereby American oncologists in private practice buy injectable drugs at wholesale, mark up the price, and then sell them retail to their patients in their offices. Under such a scheme, a private oncologist's office also operates as a pharmacy. The doctors who participate in this practice have an economic incentive to choose one drug over another because they receive greater reimbursement for one drug than another.[364]

Since oncologists can purchase these agents at prices lower than the amounts that Medicare and private insurance companies compensate for them, they get to pocket the difference. As I shall show, the mark-up has historically been *as high as 86 percent.*[365]

The public did not know about the existence of the Chemotherapy Concession until 1999. That year, at a Medicare Advisory Panel meeting in Baltimore, a gastroenterologist complained that the government had reduced his reimbursement rate for colonoscopies from $400 to $108. All the doctors in his internal medicine group were hurting, he continued, except for the two medical oncologists, whom he said were making a fortune running their in-office retail pharmacies.[366] This offhand remark alerted the world to the fact that oncologists were selling drugs at a profit in their offices.

At the *Medical News Today* Web site, patient advocate Gregory D. Pawelski, who lost his wife to ovarian cancer, describes the process thus:

"Not only do the medical oncologists have complete logistical, administrative, marketing and financial control of the process, they also control the knowledge of the process. The result is that the medical oncologist selects the product, selects the vendor, decides the markup, conceals details of the transaction to the degree they wish, and delivers the product on their own terms including time, place and modality."[367]

The Chemotherapy Concession potentially harms patients in three ways:

It creates a potential conflict of interest for oncologists, who can derive a considerable portion of their income from the sale of particular drugs;

It may expose patients to drugs with unsubstantiated benefits, since the choice is influenced by the doctor's profits rather than proven efficacy; and

It may add to the patient's direct medical costs or deplete his or her insurance benefits or coverage on futile drugs.

The existence of the Chemotherapy Concession as a source of profit can influence an oncologist's prescribing decisions. Prof. Mireille Jacobson, then of the University of California, Irvine, *et al.*, published a study in *Health Affairs*, entitled "Does reimbursement influence chemo-

176/ CUSTOMIZED CANCER TREATMENT

therapy treatment for cancer patients?"[368] The answer was in the affirmative. This form of reimbursement prompted some oncologists to utilize more expensive drugs that offered better mark-ups compared to less expensive or generic drugs. This 2006 study also found that for breast cancer patients, each dollar's worth of increase in a physician's reimbursement resulted in the use of chemotherapeutic drugs that cost the patient an additional $23.00.

The author states:

"Although reimbursement seems to have little effect on the primary decision to administer palliative chemotherapy to patients with advanced solid tumors, *it appears to affect the choice of drugs used.* Providers who were more generously reimburse... prescribed more costly chemotherapy regimens to metastatic breast, colorectal, and lung cancer patients"[369] (emphasis added).

This is to be expected, when the doctor him- or herself profits from the use of one drug over another.

Neil Love, MD, has meticulously analyzed the effects of the Chemotherapy Concession on doctor's prescribing habits. Love runs a company called Research to Practice, which analyzes doctors' therapeutic decision-making. In a 2005 report, *Patterns of Care*, he showed that the Medicare reform act (MMA) had not succeeded in reducing oncologist's incentives to prescribe based on profitability.

The Chemotherapy Concession applies only to drugs that are injected or infused, not to orally administered drugs. Love showed that for the first line chemotherapy of metastatic breast cancer in a 57-year-old woman, 88 percent of academic center-based oncologists prescribed the orally administered drug Xeloda (capecitabine). They do this because these academic doctors do *not* derive any personal profit by prescribing any particular kind of chemotherapy. Conversely, only 13 percent of them prescribed an infusional drug, such as paclitaxel (Taxol), and none of them prescribed the expensive, but highly remunerative drug docetaxel (Taxotere).

By contrast, however, with community-based oncologists (who may derive personal profit by administering infusions of chemotherapy), the picture was almost entirely reversed. Of these doctors in private practice only 20 percent said they would prescribe the *orally* administered drug (capecitabine), while 75 percent of them prescribed *infusional* drugs, and a whopping 29 percent prescribed the expensive and highly remunerative Taxotere.[370,371]

Although the Jacobson study did not conclude that chemotherapy itself was prescribed because of the Chemotherapy Concession, Love's report contradicts that conclusion. Thus, when asked if they would give chemotherapy to a 75-year-old woman with a 1.2 centimeter, node negative, estrogen receptor-positive tumor, 27 percent of the oncologists in private practice cent of the oncologists in private practice said they would, while zero percent of the academic breast cancer experts agreed! (The benefit of chemotherapy in this situation is approximately 1.5 percent alive at 10 years as a result of the treatment.)[372]

According to the *New York Times:*

"Some physicians say that cancer doctors responded to Medicare's change by performing additional treatments that got them the best reimbursements, whether or not the treatments benefited patients. Those doctors also say that Medicare's reimbursement policies are responsible."[373]

Medicare has tried to crack down on oncologists' windfall profits from prescribing particular drugs. In the late 1990s, investigations by the Department of Health and Human Services, the Department of Justice, and the House Committee on Energy and Commerce revealed that Medicare payments for chemotherapy were much higher than physicians' costs of acquiring these drugs.[374,375]

Oncologists, they said, were buying these drugs for well below the average wholesale price (AWP). In 1999, the average discount to physicians was 12 to 30 percent below the AWP but reached as high as 86 percent.[376]

One of the purposes of the Medicare Prescription Drug, Improvement, and Modernization Act (MMA) of 2003 was to alter the structure of chemotherapy reimbursements, so that physicians would be paid the manufacturers' average sales price (ASP) plus just six percent and an administrative fee. It was thus supposed to reign in the Chemotherapy Concession, at least as far as the federal government was concerned.

But this Medicare "crackdown" did not stop some doctors from continuing to profit beyond the six percent markup, as they continued to lobby Medicare officials and members of Congress to raise the prices that the government pays for drugs, again in order to increase their own profits.

The American Society of Clinical Oncology (ASCO) was a major player in these negotiations. ASCO maintains a permanent lobbying presence on Capitol Hill. In 2005, according to an ASCO press release, "the Society provided Congress...its perspective on several key issues, including Medicare reimbursement for chemotherapy drugs and services...."[377] In 2009 it was represented by Bryan Cave, LLP, which also represents many health care organizations on Capitol Hill.[378]

According to an industry newsletter *Oncology Times*, ASCO itself was involved in lobbying efforts to preserve Average Wholesale Price (AWP) overpayments, which are a key component of the Chemotherapy Concession:

"Lobbyists working for the American Society of Clinical Oncology have their thumbs firmly planted in the legislative dam holding back the deluge of law makers intent on wiping out average wholesale price (AWP)....

"The bill [the one supported by ASCO, ed.] also aims to keep much of the Medicare funds that now flow to oncologists through AWP flowing in the same direction."[379]

According to the *New York Times*, "cancer doctors billed about $4.4 billion for chemotherapy and anemia medications in 2005, down from $5.6 billion in 2004, with Medicare covering 80 percent of the bills in each year. *The difference mostly represented profit that doctors had made on the drugs*" (emphasis added).

So there are still billions of dollars involved in these decisions, enough to make many doctors quite wealthy in the process. Medicare, and insurance plans in general, reimburse physicians for chemotherapy drugs at rates that greatly exceeded physicians' own costs for those drugs.

2010 Jacobson Study

A 2010 study provided further evidence that some oncologists continue to prescribe chemotherapy based on their own financial reward rather than the medical needs of their patients. The study, also by Mireille Jacobson *et al.*, showed that when the US Congress tried to reduce Medicare spending in 2003, some oncologists responded by treating a greater number of patients with more expensive drugs to make up for this lost income.[380]

"Many doctors ended up prescribing chemotherapy for more of their patients, to make up for lower prices," commented Reed Abelson, who follows this issue for the *New York Times.* In some cases, doctors bought drugs at 20 percent below Medicare's reimbursement rate. This generated "large sums" (ibid.) because of the difference between the wholesale and the retail (i.e., Medicare) prices.

The authors of the article in *Health Affairs* analyzed the records of over 200,000 US lung cancer patients treated between 2003 and 2005. Contrary to expectations, when the Medicare cuts went into effects, doctors wound up giving more extensive (and expensive) treatments.

Before the law went into effect, 16.5 percent of such patients received chemotherapy. After the law went into effect this rose to 18.9 percent of patients. Although the authors only analyzed lung cancer, this 2.4 percent difference could be considerable, especially if applied to a substantial portion of the 1,529,460 Americans that are predicted to develop cancer in 2010, according to the American Cancer Society (ACS).

"In sum, far from limiting access," the changes under the law "actually increased the likelihood that lung cancer patients received chemotherapy," said Jacobson.

The authors focused on lung cancer because of the various treatment options for that disease, some of which are considerably more expensive than others. They found that doctors frequently switched drugs to choose the more expensive options. There was, for instance, an increased use of docetaxel (Taxotere), a drug for which oncologist get reimbursed about $2,500 per patient per month.

"The financial incentive seemed to have an effect where there's not strong evidence or more than one equally good treatment option," said Craig C. Earle, MD, of Toronto, one of the study authors.

Oncologists reacted by treating a greater number of such patients because they had been making so much money under the old system, Prof. Joseph P. Newhouse of Harvard University, another co-author, told the *Times*. "These markups were a substantial portion of their income."[381]

The bottom line was that some oncologists in private practice made crucial treatment decisions not based on medical necessity but on what is most profitable for them-selves.

No one should begrudge oncologists high salaries. They are skilled professionals, who deserve our support and respect. However, the Chemotherapy Concession introduces a temptation to oncologists in private practice to prescribe according to their economic interests rather than the medical needs of their patients. This has no scientific or moral justification. Congress still needs to thoroughly investigate and fix this problem.

Matter of Rebate

In addition to the Chemotherapy Concession there is the matter of rebates. According to a 2007 editorial in the *New York Times*, the sale of expensive oncology-related drugs (Aranesp, Epogen and Procrit) "has been propelled" by two companies "paying out hundreds of millions of dollars in so-called rebates.

Doctors typically buy the drugs from the companies, get reimbursed for much of the cost by Medicare and private insurers, and on top of that get these rebates based on the amount they have purchased."[382]

"There's pretty good evidence at this point," said Richard Deyo, MD, professor of medicine at the University of Washington and an expert on health care spending, "that there are plenty of patients for whom there's little hope, who are terminally ill, whom chemotherapy is not going to help, who get chemotherapy."[383]

Ari Straus, MD, chief operating officer of Aurora Healthcare Consulting, which helps doctors increase their profits, said Medicare's changes had squeezed oncologists. "Five years ago, many physicians were earning over $1 million per year on drug sales alone," according to Mr. Straus.[384]

"People go where the money is, and you'd like to believe it's different in medicine, but it's really no different in medicine," said Robert Geller, MD, who worked as an oncologist in private practice from 1996 to 2005. "When you start thinking of oncology as a business, then all these decisions make sense."[385]

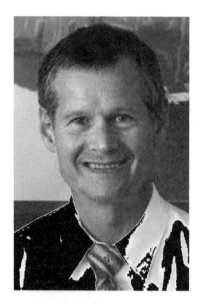

Larry Weisenthal, MD, PhD, of
Weisenthal Cancer Group

VII. OTHER FORMS OF THE TEST

We shall now turn out attention to some alternate forms of the Test, which possibly could represent the future of the field.

A major practical impediment to the use of the Test is that patients must have access to a fresh piece of tumor for analysis. But in Europe, there are laboratories that claim to perform the Test in the absence of fresh tumor samples. These laboratories (see Appendix B) claim to be able to conduct *in vitro* tests for chemotherapy on circulating tumor cells (CTCs) that are isolated from the blood sample of a patient and then to analyze these cells for their drug susceptibilities.

This idea is very attractive since it can analyze not just tumors or tumor effusion materials, but, in some cases, from peripheral blood as well. Some even claim to be able to find CTCs in relatively early stages of the disease. This would indeed be what one scientist called the "Holy Grail" of oncology, since it would eliminate the difficulty of obtaining fresh biopsy samples to repeatedly perform the Test on fresh operative or biopsy specimens.

Pachmann Laboratory

In Appendix B, I list three such laboratories. In my opinion, the most impressive is the Laboratory for Specific Immunohematology and Gene Diagnostics of Bayreuth, Germany. The Pachmann laboratory claims to be able to routinely isolate CTCs from the blood, bone marrow and other bodily fluids of patients who have relatively early stages of cancer.

The Pachmann laboratory is headed by Ulrich Pachmann, MD and utilizes the work of his wife, Katharina M. Pachmann, MD, and her colleagues, at the Friedrich Schiller University of Jena. Katharina Pachmann and her academic colleagues have published a number of provocative papers on CTCs and the testing process.

The Pachmanns use their proprietary MAINTRAC™ analysis (US patent #7615358), which they describe as an "extremely sensitive and specific approach" to quantifying minimal numbers of circulating tumor cells (CTCs) in blood and bone marrow in patients with solid tumors.[386]

The Pachmanns advocate using "extremely sensitive techniques" that are "easily applied to peripheral blood samples" to detect the progression of cancer at virtually every stage of the disease.[387] For example, K. Pachmann has monitored CTCs throughout the course of neoadjuvant chemotherapy (i.e., chemotherapy given before surgery in order to shrink the tumor and make it more amenable to removal).[388]

She has also monitored CTCs in the course of adjuvant therapy, i.e., therapy given after the surgical removal of the tumor. Typically, oncologists do not expect there to be CTCs in such a situation, although Pachmann has reported finding them in a surprising number of cases.

What is more, their presence and number can supposedly serve as good prognosticators:

"Nineteen patients with a decline or no change in number of CETC [i.e., CTCs] showed no relapse whereas six patients with a more than ten-fold increase had five distant and one local relapse, indicating that the dynamic of CETC in the individual patient is predictive of outcome."[389]

One of Pachmann's most provocative claims is that she can detect "circulating epithelial cells in 92 percent of breast and lung cancer patients."[390]

She studied 25 consecutive *non-metastatic* primary breast cancer patients who were receiving adjuvant chemotherapy. CTCs were assayed before and after the second cycle of chemotherapy. CTCs showed a decline, no change or a minor increase in 15 patients, of whom 14 remained in complete remission. But of ten patients who showed an increase in CTCs by the end of therapy, four relapsed. Her conclusion was that the response of CTCs to therapy was "an independent predictive marker for relapse."[391]

It is very interesting that CTCs (at least in Pachmann's tests) could be used so accurately to predict the outcome of adjuvant chemotherapy. But more astonishing is the fact that, in her work, CTCs are detected so routinely in women who clearly do not have what would conventionally be called advanced disease. In fact, Pachmann has made the provocative claim that surgery routinely *drives* epithelial cells (including presumably cancer cells) into the blood circulation.

As odd (and frightening) as this sounds, she is hardly alone in this belief. In 2004, a team based at the University of Texas Southwestern Medical Center, Dallas, also reported finding CTCs in 13 of 36 (36 percent) of breast cancer patients a full 7 to 22 years after their successful mastectomies. They were without any evidence of disease and would conventionally be considered cured, but they clearly had dormant breast cancer.[392]

At the 2005 meeting of the American Association for Cancer Research (AACR), *Oncology Times* reported:

"Evidence is mounting that these cells arise very early in disease progression....The data support the hypotheses that tumor-cell dissemination is an early event and that it increases with the aggressiveness of the tumor."[393]

There was also a similar study of the bone marrow of men with "clinically localized" prostate cancer at the University of Washington Medical School and the Fred Hutchinson Cancer Research Center. But in these so-called early stage patients *disseminated* epithelial (presumably cancer) cells were detected in 56 percent of prostatectomy patients, and prostate-specific antigen (PSA)-positive disseminated tumor cells were also detected in 31 percent of patients. By contrast, they were found in 9 percent of the aspirates of men without a diagnosis of cancer.

In a 2009 follow-up, this same group reported:

"Approximately 70 percent of men undergoing radical prostatectomy had DTC [disseminated tumor cell, ed.] detected in their bone marrow prior to surgery, suggesting that these cells escape early in the disease. Although preoperative DTC status does not correlate with pathologic risk factors, persistence of DTC after radical prostatectomy in NED patients was an independent predictor of recurrence."[394]

The idea of detecting tumor cells in the circulating blood of patients with cancer is no longer controversial. A turning point came in January 2004, when the FDA granted permission to Veridex, Inc. (a branch of the giant Johnson & Johnson pharmaceutical company) to market its CellSearch™ kit for diagnostic purposes in colorectal cancer. The FDA has since extended this approval to metastatic breast and prostate cancer.

In September 2009, the NCI held a conference of 500 researchers on this general topic.[395] As NCI's weekly *Cancer Bulletin* reported:

"At Stanford University, researchers are asking whether the analysis of CTCs can match patients and drugs early in treatment. The team will profile certain genes in CTCs using blood drawn from men with prostate cancer before and after they receive an experimental drug. As the trial progresses, it will be clear who the responders are, and the researchers will then look for associations with CTC gene profiles."[396]

This is similar in important ways to the approach of the Pachmanns and a few other European laboratories. So the idea that there are CTCs present and detectable in the blood, blood marrow and other bodily fluids of patients with less advanced cancers (or no evidence of cancer) is becoming increasingly accepted.

Pachmann also used the MAINTRAC analysis to monitor the number of epithelial cells before, 30 minutes, 60 minutes, three and seven days after surgery and during subsequent follow-up.

One of her key findings: "Circulating epithelial cells were already present before surgery in all patients."[397]

These values started to rise during the following three to four days *up to thousand fold* in 85 percent of the treated patients "in spite of complete resection of the tumor with tumor free margins in all patients."[398]

In many cases, the number of CTCs subsequently declined, but in 58 percent of cases the numbers remained above pre-surgery levels until the onset of chemotherapy. In women who did not get adjuvant treatment because they were considered at "low risk," the CTC numbers remained elevated for up to three years. The authors surprising conclusions are as follows:

"Frequently before but regularly during surgery of breast cancer, epithelial cells are mobilized into circulation....Cells can remain in the circulation over long times. Such cells may remain 'dormant' but might settle and grow into metastases, if they find appropriate conditions, even after years."[399]

What remains unclear is how well this test performs in terms of its sensitivity and specificity in predicting the most beneficial forms of chemotherapy. Dr. Pachmann has written: "One of the main advantages of our method is the possibility to test the sensitivity of these cells to the chemotherapeutic agents planned for treatment."[400] She has also sent me a poster presentation at the 2009 San Antonio Breast Cancer Symposium. This details the methods used, but provides only three correlations.[401]

While Pachmann's ideas are provocative, I feel it would be necessary to see a clear-cut comparison of test results achieved with the MAINTRAC system vis-a-vis the live tumor sample-based forms of chemosensitivity testing in order to make a meaningful comparison.

Biofocus

Another European laboratory that provides a chemosensitivity assessment of CTCs is Biofocus. This was founded as Relab in 1991 and is presently located in Recklinghausen, Germany. The researchers there could not give me any detailed information on either the sensitivity or the specificity of its test. They did provide me with a paper by seven German scientists that contains some information.[402]

This paper describes "novel diagnostic techniques to identify minimal tumor cells." The main technique sdescribed in the article is the so-called GeneStick™ cancer sensor. This allegedly measures the expression level of "150 drug-related genes [that] covers practically the entire spectrum of antitumor therapy." They describe it as "the first step towards a personalized cancer treatment."

Dr. Lothar Prix of Biofocus further stated:

"We have not done huge studies, but a study of Dr Scheller‡‡‡‡‡ from Leonardis Clinic has shown predictive value of our analysis. Also, many of the clinics using our testing for a long time now consider it useful."[403]

What Dr. Prix apparently refers to is a table in an article, "The Predictive Potency of Drug Targeting in Disseminated Micrometastases." This is a list of eight cases (3 breast cancer, 1 ovarian, 2 colorectal, 1 stomach, 1 thymoma) and attempts to correlate the results of Bio-Focus's testing with clinical outcomes.

---

‡‡‡‡‡ Albert Scheller, MD, was long-time medical director of the Leonardis Klinik, Bad Heilbrunn, Germany. He died of a heart attack in Las Vegas, Nevada, on August 29, 2005. The Leonardis Klinik, now closed, also used the services of the Pachmann laboratory.

The authors claim that when four of these patients were treated according to the results of molecular testing,§§§§§§ there was "improved clinical outcome" in all four cases, whereas in the other four cases that did not follow molecular testing there was "reduced outcome."

I find it impossible to interpret such a small number of cases published in a journal of undetermined origin. What are we to make, for instance, of breast cancer case #2, whose cells were found to be sensitive to the drug methotrexate but not to 5-FU, yet who was apparently treated with both drugs and then had a partial response? How are we to know that it was methotrexate, and not 5-FU, that conveyed the therapeutic benefit?

Similarly, what about ovarian case #4, who was found to be sensitive to cyclophosphamide but resistant to gemcitabine? This patient was then given both drugs but passed away. How are we to know that this was a failure of one drug and not the other? To be generous, one might conclude that this table represents eight correlations of tests with outcomes. But this is a very small number on which to base life-and-death decisions, especially when we consider that there are at least 4,263 correlations

---

§§§§§§ The patient with colorectal cancer was treated on two separate occasions, with different drugs and different outcomes, and is thus counted in the authors' calculations as two cases.

supporting the sensitivity and specificity of the Test that utilizes samples of viable tumor tissue. I would need to see a much fuller presentation of correlations before I could believe in the validity of this form of testing.

The Greek Laboratory

In northwestern Greece, Dr. Ioannis Papasotiriou runs the modern and well-equipped Research Genetic Cancer Center (RGCC). This is the laboratory used by many central European complementary and alternative clinics and an increasing number of American doctors as well.

Papasotiriou and his colleagues use a variety of techniques to analyze tumor and blood specimens. These include some of the older tests, including clonogenic, ATP-TCA, MTT and SRB assays.

They are best known, however, for isolating CTCs from cancer patients' blood and growing tumor cell cultures in 96-well plates. Into each well they then add a different chemotherapeutic drug. There are four steps to their analysis:

The isolation of sample cancer cells and the development of primary cultures.

Introduction of a different chemotherapeutic drug into each well.

Testing of the genes of the cancer cells by a microarray analysis. They then use various techniques to probe for a variety of genes, such as topo-I, p27 and p53.

Verification of the genetic analysis by small-scale viability testing of the cultures.

This process differs from the techniques used at most chemosensitivity laboratories in the United States that use programmed cell death as their primary end point. At such labs, there is a general policy against *growing* or *manipulating* the tumor cells in any way.

In other words, when one is looking for programmed cell death-related events, which mirror the effect of drugs on living tumors, cells are generally not grown or amplified in any way. Also, in the main type of the Test discussed in this book there is no emphasis placed on the presence or absence of particular genes, as in the Greek lab.

The main thing that matters in the classic chemosensitivity laboratories is the occurrence of PCD in cells that come into contact with the candidate therapeutic agents. Genetic analysis takes us into an entirely different realm, one that is far removed from the subject of this book and what most people know as the Test.

The Greek laboratory also states at its Web site that they can isolate CTCs from venous blood in cases of cancer when the "disease is systematic in the stage IIi and above." In other words, they claim that in stage II the disease can already be systemic and that wayward cancer cells are circulating in the bloodstream. In earlier stages they too require a tissue sample packed in saline with the antibiotic streptomycin to prevent bacterial contamination.

Questions About Isolating CTCs

From the point of view of standard chemosensitivity testing, however, there are many questions about the accuracy of this sort of testing of circulating tumor cells.

Again, the "Holy Grail" aspect of these tests is so important that their claims should not be ignored. If they are accurate, then a new milestone has truly been reached in cancer treatment and no cancer clinic should be without this test. On the other hand, if they are inaccurate then patients are being misdirected to a less-than-optimal treatment program.

One question is how any of these European laboratories can aggregate a sufficient number of cancer cells to make accurate determinations. In their successful 2009 US patent application, the Pachmann team states:

"Detectable tumor cells in the peripheral blood are present only in extremely small numbers."[404] This then precludes allowing a sufficient number of cells to simply incubate for a few days in the presence of chemotherapeutic agents.

But, according to Nagourney, performing a genomic or proteomic analysis of a relatively small number of isolated cancer cells (such as the Stanford laboratory, cited above, also hopes to do) cannot yield the same quality information as actually subjecting living cells to chemotherapeutic agents.

It also begs the question of whether or not genomic or proteomic analysis of this sort can accurately predict which drugs will work and which will not. This is far from certain, and in any case cannot be classified as a form of chemosensitivity testing.

And what exactly *are* these CTCs? They are free floating cancer cells that can remain in isolation from a tumor for over 20 years (presumably in the bone marrow "homing organ"[405]). What are the implications of this survival for clinical practice? What is the relationship of such long-lasting cells to the tumor cells that need to be attacked through the tested substances?

Also, there is a question of heterogeneity, i.e., the fact that tumors in the body are genetically variable. This is a problem for the Test, as indicated above. But it may be a particular problem for these CTC-based tests, since it has not been established what the relationship is between circulating tumor cells and primary tumors or their already established metastases.

There is now evidence that "the gene expression profile of the metastatic lesion can be different compared to that of the primary" breast cancer.[406] For instance, the status of the marker HER/2-neu in CTCs sometimes differs from that of the original primary tumor, which would point to different prescriptions for the drug Herceptin (trastuzumab).[407]

There is a credible amount of data that CTCs can be isolated from various bodily fluids, including circulating blood, in a surprisingly large number of cancer patients. The number of cells discovered in these tests is also turning out to be a good prognosticator of how well (empiric) treatments are working. But less certain is the ability to use these CTCs as the basis of chemosensitivity assays.

According to Cristofanilli and Mendelsohn:

"Clinical trials testing correlations between gene status data obtained from CTCs before treatment and the responses of patients to various therapeutic regimens might lead to diagnostic tests that can select the therapy most likely to be effective for an individual patient."[408]

This is of course the great hope. I am not implying that this approach will not work. I am only saying that allsuch approaches (which are similar to the approach already pursued by the European laboratories mentioned above) are far less documented in their actual predictive value than the established chemosensitivity tests.

The European CTC-based laboratories have a great idea. In particular, if CTCs can be isolated earlier in the disease process than is generally recognized (as Katharina Pachmann has postulated), and if these CTCs can then be analyzed to differentiate between effective and ineffective drugs, then this is outstanding work.

At the present time, in my opinion, this remains a tantalizing but unproven proposition. The level of documentation of the sensitivity and specificity of the drug recommendations that are generated by this procedure has to be culled from various papers, but has never been the subject of a single peer-reviewed article.

Thus, in my opinion, it remains questionable whether one should entrust one's future treatment (and possibly one's life) to such an uncertain course, especially if more conventional chemosensitivity testing on a live cancer sample is feasible. For that reason, whenever possible, I would try to obtain living tissue for the Test rather than rely on the less documented genetic analysis of peripheral blood.

Genetic Testing

The isolation of CTCs raises the question of how accurate an analysis of genetic material is in finding the peculiarities of a tumor and guiding future treatment.

Christofanilli and Mendelsohn describe this in the following glowing terms:

"The sophisticated analysis of single cells offered by application of novel technologies has opened the possibility of a new era in the development of more "tailored" and personalized therapies."[409]

This is an amazing statement. These distinguished authors are speaking of isolating and analyzing *single* cancer cells! This sort of genomic approach has begun, with tests for the HER2-neu gene, the BRCA 1 and 2 genes, and the Oncotype DX test on biopsy samples. It is certainly going to thrive in the present era of "personalized medicine," with its emphasis on genetic testing.

I do not know if testing of this sort will yield important results for the majority of common cancers, as the director of the National Institutes of Health (NIH), Francis S. Collins, MD and many other medical leaders fervently believe.

What I find irksome, however, is that an established and very good technology, the Test, which could be put into wide-scale practice right now, is being ignored, while all emphasis is put on the unsubstantiated supposition that common cancers may someday be detected and cured through analysis at a genetic level of a small number of cells or even a single wayward cell.

Genetic or immunohistochemical testing as it currently exists generally examines dead tissue that is preserved in paraffin or formalin. How predictive is that likely to be of the behavior of living cells in spontaneously formed colonies or microspheres? Can DNA tests describe the complex behavior of living cancer cells in response to the injury they receive from particular forms of chemotherapy? One must always bear in mind the difference between living and dead tissues.

Some molecular tests do in fact utilize living cells, but generally of *individual cancer cells in suspension,* sometimes derived from tumors and sometimes from circulating tumor cells (CTCs). This may sound innovative and high tech, but scientists should remember that this too was tried years ago through the human clonogenic assay and was found to be of limited value.

Customized Medicine?

For the vast majority of people, cancer treatment, as it is presently administered, is not customized. Treatment protocols are based on the results of large randomized clinical trials, generally performed at NCI-designated comprehensive cancer centers (CCCs). In these trials, and in the protocols that emerge from them, there is no room for matching the individual patients' cancer cells with the drugs given. What patients get instead are myriad variations on run-of-the-mill drug combinations, which Weisenthal justifiably calls "lowest-common-denominator chemotherapy."[410] This practice is based on the illusion of the average patient, a fictional person who does not actually exist.[411]

Top leaders of the medical profession have spoken eloquently about how they intend to transform cancer treatment based on the individual characteristics of real patients. In August 2008, the former NCI director John E. Niederhuber, MD, wrote an editorial, "The Dawn of Personalized Oncology," on this topic. The overarching slogan of the 2009 annual meeting of the American Society of Clinical Oncology (ASCO) was also "Personalized Cancer Medicine."[412]

Slogans of this sort are catching on. In October 2009, Ohio State University's Center for Personalized Health Care hosted a national conference on the topic of "Transforming Health Care Through Personalized Medicine."[413]

In late 2009, upon exiting Port Columbus International Airport, I was astonished to see a gigantic billboard promoting individualized patient care at the nearby James Cancer Center. A woman who is totally bald, presumably as a result of her chemotherapy, explains to passing travelers: "I have a team of experts who are focused on treating just one type of cancer—mine."

In 2010, NIH director Francis S. Collins, MD authored a book subtitled *DNA and the Revolution in Personalized Medicine*.[414] At first, this may seem like a ringing endorsement of the Test. But actually the present-day conception of "customized" or "personalized medicine" coming from our medical leaders has *nothing to do* with the Test described in this book. In fact, it is a cooptation of the fundamental appeal of the Test, without any of the substance.

The medical leaders who are now promoting this new 'personalized' medicine have no intention whatsoever of revitalizing the chemosensitivity testing program, at NCI or elsewhere, much less of supporting the work going on at the independent laboratories doing that work. They are going off in a different direction, genomics, which 'personalizes' treatment based on the genetic peculiarities of the patient, rather than the unique reaction of each patient's cancer cells to an array of possible drugs.

Dr. Niederhuber, for instance, discusses:

Target identification through high-throughput screening;

Chemical characterization and structural design optimization at the molecular target interaction;

Testing in genetically engineered mice; and

Design of mechanisms for monitoring *in vivo* activity (in living beings).

At the end of this complicated process, he says, comes translation of these research results to man.[415] What is wrong with this picture? In his three-and-a-half page editorial there is not a single mention of the Test.

It is as if 50 years of determined effort by scores of outstanding researchers in dozens of laboratories around the world had simply fallen into a black hole.

What Niederhuber *et al.* are talking about is genetic testing (perhaps based on an analysis of the total human genome of each individual) followed by the administration of drugs based on the perceived genetic peculiarities of the individual in question.

One can easily see the appeal of this sort of automated testing. I am not saying it will not work, since it is essentially untried. But at the present time it is largely an unexplored area, more sci-fi than science. Whatever its ultimate merit it should not be counterpoised to the mature and successful field of actually existing chemosensitivity assays.

There is currently a lot of blue-sky speculation about what the personalized medicine of the future might look like. But if one were sincerely interested in individualizing medicine, why not start right now with the technology that already exists to do that—third generation, PCD-based chemosensitivity assays?

Perhaps the answer is that to do so one would have to confront not just the medical prejudices that exist against the Test (mainly as a result of the flawed ASCO evaluation) but various obstacles devised by the medical insurance industry, the clinical trial establishment, and other enterprises that may not like the idea of designing treatment protocols based on laboratory testing.

So acceptance of such tests faces daunting obstacles in defenders of the status quo, of whom there are many. I have no doubt that in the end the truth about the Test will emerge and that this technology will greatly improve the outcome of chemotherapy and other forms of cancer treatment. I am equally certain that this will not happen without a concerted struggle that will involve those most interested in a successful outcome, the patients.

VIII. CONCLUSIONS

Finally, I want to discuss some of the broader implications of the Test to the world of cancer medicine. For instance, the use of the Test has so far mainly been limited to chemotherapy. However, there are several other applications that could be explored once this primary usage is more widely accepted.

The Test and CAM

Another exciting prospect is the revolutionary potential of the Test in the field of complementary and alternative medicine (CAM). At the present time, there are many treatments of natural origin that have been proposed as candidates for cancer therapy. These are widely used both as self-help techniques and in CAM clinics. Some of these may have great value, although most are inadequately researched or documented.

We should remember that about one-quarter of all chemotherapeutic agents have a natural origin. This includes such important drugs as the taxanes (ultimately derived from the Pacific Yew tree), the Vinca alkaloids (from the Madagascar periwinkle), bryostatins (from the marine organism, *Bugula neritina*) as well as cisplatin and other derivatives of the mineral platinum. Many other such agents are waiting in the wings, their development held up by the great expense and difficulty of the drug approval process.

Despite the lack of clarity on the safety and efficacy of these agents, at the present time many patients self-medicate with a wide variety of these natural approaches. How commonly? A survey by the National Institutes of Health (NIH) found that 63 percent of adult cancer patients (who were participating in clinical trials) used at least one CAM therapy, with an average use of two such treatments per patient.[416]

The number of CAM users may actually be higher, since these patients do not necessarily tell their oncologists about such usage, for fear of an unsympathetic reaction. Those who use such treatments tend to be highly positive about the experience. "Patients unanimously believed that these complementary therapies helped to improve their quality of life," NIH researchers reported.[417]

All too commonly, however, patients and their loved ones are uncertain which CAM treatments to use. This can lead to nihilistic despair at the prospect of finding effective agents or, conversely, a tendency to throw "the kitchen sink" of complementary and alternative approaches at the tumor. In other words, there is little *objective* guidance into what is likely to work or not work for any particular case.

Chemosensitivity testing, when applied to CAM, would provide a similar service as it does to chemotherapy, and could become the ultimate guide to choosing treatments that are likely to work and avoiding those that do not, at least in terms of causing programmed cell death.

The acceptance of the Test for chemotherapy would therefore be likely to similarly revolutionize the practice of CAM.

At the present time, none of the American chemosensitivity laboratories routinely screens natural agents. (A few of them will screen such agents if the patient explicitly requests it and provides a sample.) The aforementioned European laboratories that provide analysis based on circulating tumor cells do routinely provide an analysis of a variety of CAM agents, but, as I have indicated, these are subject to various caveats.

There is no reason that others could not and would not do this sort of CAM testing if the Test were made routine. Certainly, not all CAM treatments work by means of stimulating PCD, but those that do could be discovered via the Test. Certain unconventional treatments would thus quite readily be shown to work in specific patients. Others might be revealed to be essentially inert at least as far as the PCD endpoints go. And some would be found to work in a small minority of cases. Thus, the Test could be a kind of Occam's razor, which could greatly simplify the present-day jumble of potential CAM treatments.

In conclusion, one of the great tragedies of our day, as far as cancer is concerned, is the near complete 'boycott' of chemosensitivity testing by the mainstream medical community. Are advocates of the Test responsible for the lack of progress in the field, including the lack of RCTs? It is sometimes assumed that they are, and that they advocate this method of testing because of their own self-interest. I find a variety of negative statements about the Test on the Web. For instance, an anonymous oncologist posted a typical such reaction at the cancertests.org Web site:

"There has never been an iota of proof that *ex vivo* drug sensitivity testing is an effective method for selecting an individual's therapy in any cancer. The only sources of enthusiasm for this concept are the companies continuing to test for profit. Continuing NCI funding for this effort after a huge expenditure, without proof of concept or new and better methods of testing would be a waste of taxpayer's money."[418]

Sometimes people who engage in this type of criticisms are themselves the beneficiaries of the status quo in cancer care. When affiliated with major institutions, such critics may even have the ability to arrange the larger, more definitive trials that they demand, while the objects of their criticism do not. In other words, the shoe is on the wrong foot.

The large institutions have failed to carry confirmatory and comparative tests of third generation chemosensitivity testing, despite the fact that authoritative sources have repeatedly pointed out the urgent necessity of doing so. Instead, they have apparently been influenced by the prejudicial ASCO review that supposedly shows the Test to be inadequately proven and therefore (by an unknown leap of logic) unworthy of further consideration.

As a result of such *ex cathedra* condemnations, investigation of the Test has ground to a halt at NCI and at the comprehensive cancer centers that it so generously supports. This lack of randomized trials (again, assuming that they are even necessary) has become a *self-fulfilling prophecy* on the part of these critics.

They demand a level of proof that only they and their well-funded colleagues could provide, knowing full well that the advocates of the Test, who direct relatively small private laboratories, long ago reached the limits of their own resources.

The Test and Radiation

An area that has been insufficiently explored is the possibility of using the Test to predict a patient's response to radiation therapy. In fact, the clonogenic assay was originally invented in the 1950s as a way of assessing the impact of radiation on tumor cell growth.[419]

The pioneering Chicago area oncologist Robert Schrek applied the Test to the field of radiation therapy. He found that people vary greatly in the susceptibility of their cells to radiation. For instance, while some patients' leukemia (CLL) cells could be destroyed with a mere two roentgens [i.e., cGys] of radiation, a few patients had cells that could withstand 1,000 roentgens. [420]

In 1992, Hinkley and Bosanquet of the Bath Cancer Research Unit researched this topic in chronic lymphocytic leukemia (CLL) and had some preliminary success.[421] They reported:

"The results of 61 CLL specimens from 40 patients [showed] profound inter-patient differences in the sensitivity of cells to radiation. Five patient specimens, which were radio-resistant *in vitro*, were from patients who were also resistant clinically to irradiation. Another patient who responded very well clinically was found to be extremely sensitive in the assay."[422]

In 1999, Comby, of the University of Caen, also observed this relationship in B-cell CLL and predicted the utility of the Test in this situation:

"In the future, a valuable clue to the selection of irradiation regimens for B-CLL patients may be the investigation of correlations between *in vitro* radiation-induced apoptosis and the *in vivo* response to radiation therapy."[423]

Despite these reports, I am unaware of any laboratory in the world that is currently offering the Test before patients undergo radiation treatment. It seems likely that wide-scale adoption of the Test for pre-screening chemotherapy would stimulate research into its possible application in radiation therapy.

The 'Holy Grail'

The Test was once hailed as the "Holy Grail" of cancer research, according to Matti S. Aapro, MD, Secretary-General Emeritus of the European Organization for the Research and Treatment of Cancer (EORTC).[424]

For decades, a reliable and universally applicable method of predicting the chemosensitivity of tumors was a top agenda item for oncology. There are over a thousand articles in the scientific literature on this topic.[425]

Robert Nagourney has projected "a future when all patients will be profiled for drug response prior to the administration of systemic therapy."[426] I too foresee a future in which every living tumor sample would be routinely analyzed for its susceptibility to (a) chemotherapy drugs, both singly and in combination; (b) anti-angiogenic agents; and (c) a variety of complementary and alternative (CAM) agents, mainly of natural origin.

These tests could be performed repeatedly, at different stages in the patient's disease. Treatment would therefore proceed hand-in-hand with testing of fresh specimens of the patient's primary tumor and metastases. This would become as routine as biopsy and histological examination of tumors is today.

This wide-scale adoption of the Test does not preclude possible validation of another kind of testing: the isolation of circulating tumor cells (CTCs) and an analysis of the genomics or proteomic features of these cells. But, in this regard, we need to heed Voltaire's famous warning and not let the great become the enemy of the good.

At the present time the clinical utility of a genomic analysis of CTC as a guide to the most effective drugs is mainly a matter of *hopeful speculation.* Confirmation of its sensitivity and specificity would truly be a wonderful development in oncology. But there are many potential stumbling blocks in its ultimate realization, whereas *the Test exists here and now.*

It is available for today's patients (if their doctors cooperate in providing viable fresh tumor specimens to chemosensitivity laboratories for testing). The Test is poised to immediately become an integrated part of the regular process of drug selection.

It is therefore ridiculous to block the implementation of a *very good test* (with about 85 percent sensitivity) because scientists believe that sometime—in the next five, ten or twenty years?—there may be an even better test available!

Yet that, essentially, is the position of the top cancer leadership, which has staked its hopes and dreams on a genomic analysis of tumor cells, but given short shrift to the very good and already available forms of the Test.

Despite its long track record of success, the Test is no longer a priority for most leaders of the War on Cancer. The quest for the Holy Grail has been sidetracked, if not outright cancelled. Or perhaps the new "Holy Grail" is a genetic analysis machine in which—as I once heard an oncologist say—doctors will drop a snippet of tumor in one end and a prescription will emerge from the other end. I wish geneticists luck in developing such a machine. But they should not ignore the fact that assays exist right now for analyzing the actual behavior of an individual's cancer cells in the presence of different chemotherapeutic agents.

In Appendix A, I give the names of the dozen or so laboratories that are pursuing the Test in the US and Europe, mostly Germany.

The evidence for the effectiveness of chemosensitivity tests is solid, extensive and positive. We have reached the point where chemosensitivity testing can be performed both *reliably* and *economically* for virtually every patient.

The adoption of the Test before initiating treatment would revolutionize oncology. One hears a great deal these days about "customized oncology." The principal way that oncology could be customized, or personalized, *today* is through implementation of the Test.

If, at the time of surgery or biopsy, a portion of every patient's tumor were kept alive and promptly sent to a competent laboratory for testing, this would usher in a new era in oncology. Treatment decisions could then be made on the basis of the individual's own tumor, not some predetermined protocol derived from clinical trials.

Yet, oddly enough, neither the cancer establishment nor the rank-and-file oncologists show any particular interest in exploring or developing such tests. They have collectively closed their minds to this development—"We tried that and it didn't work." Some people accuse the developers of such tests of not providing the kind of proof required by modern medicine, or of being premature in their enthusiasm for their own specialty.[427]

But the fact is that many oncologists remain unaware of the potential value of such testing and in fact denigrate its use, often without exhibiting any awareness of the long and increasingly positive scientific basis of support.

The central mystery of the Test is therefore why more oncologists don't make use of it.

Can the Test be improved further? Of course. In any dynamically evolving area of science, innovations happen all the time. But some forms of the Test available right now are perfectly adequate for the task and should be widely and immediately utilized on live biopsy samples.

The average cancer patient is not told about their existence, much less their effectiveness at finding better drugs. In fact, should they stumble across its existence, they may even be subjected to a rude and ignorant tirade, such as I described at the start of this book.

Reevaluation of the Test

The rejection of the Test is a tragic mistake on the part of mainstream oncology. Appeals to the cancer community to re-evaluate the Test have not led to any appreciable progress. It is therefore time for those who truly care about making cancer treatment more effective, affordable and humane to take their case to the general public.

I am not recommending that they stir up populist anger against the oncology profession. But the broad public, including cancer patients, needs to be informed of the long and tortured struggle to gain acceptance for the Test.

Informed patients and their caregivers, along with concerned members of the medical profession, should petition Medicare/Medicaid, Blue Cross/Blue Shield and other health insurers to demand that they fully compensate for the Test when it is performed at nationally licensed and accredited oncology laboratories, such as those listed in Appendix A.

The negative judgment of the 2004 ASCO panel needs to be reversed. It is essential to recognize that the panel constructed its evaluation on a framework provided by the health insurance industry, used a biased methodology, and employed out-dated thinking. The new ASCO evaluators must include scientists who have actual experience researching and performing modern tests using programmed cell death (PCD) as the main endpoint. The clonogenic and other earlier tests must be recognized as irrelevant to the current situation.

These needn't even be further discussed, considered, or evaluated. To do otherwise is to get mired down in 'refuting' the irrelevant precursors of the modern field of apoptosis-based chemosensitivity testing.

We must remember that the FDA commonly approves chemotherapeutic agents of dubious safety and efficacy, for which insurers then pay large amounts of money.

For example, in September 2009 the FDA approved the drug pralatrexate (Folotyn) for the treatment of peripheral T-cell lymphoma.[428] The charge for this drug is $30,000 per month and could reach a total of $126,000 during each course of treatment. [429]

Despite that, Folotyn has never been shown to extend patients' survival, only to temporarily shrink some tumors.[430] In 2010 the FDA approved a dendritic cell-based vaccine, Provenge (sipuleucil), which will cost $93,000 for a course of three infusions. But this treatment extends life on average by only 4.1 months.[431]

the Test is better founded than most of the treatments approved by FDA. Yet it continues to be stonewalled by the oncologist profession, represented by ASCO, and by the insurance industry and regulatory authorities. This seems like gross favoritism towards the pharmaceutical industry on the part of FDA. A level playing field is the minimal requirement if more effective techniques are ever going to succeed in their struggle with better-funded competitors. It is the responsibility of the federal government to assure that level playing field.

The cost of the Test, at the laboratories listed in Appendix A, varies from $445 (at Cell Biolabs, Inc.) to $3,500 for an entire panel of drugs at some other laboratories.

The total cost of the Test is therefore, at most, *1/36th of the cost of a single course of a single drug, Folotyn.* Yet, ironically, the Test could reduce the excessive use of Folotyn (as well as other exorbitant and ineffective drugs) since chemosensitivity testing could readily rule out its use in patients for whom it is unlikely to work.

Thus, by agreeing to pay for the Test, insurance companies could actually *save* a lot of money that is currently being wasted on drugs that are used in situations in which they are unlikely to work.

It is odd that medical insurance companies will pay outrageous amounts of money for ineffective products of Big Pharma, but refuse to pay for an economical measure such as the Test.

Refusing to pay for the Test may therefore seem to be against the economic interests of the insurers. This is certainly true, but in their refusal these companies are being characteristically shortsighted, looking only to this quarter's bottom line, without considering the long-term financial (not to mention medical) benefits of compensating for the Test to cancer patients.

In the long run, timely chemosensitivity assays would lead to *major cost savings* for insurance companies, as well as better outcomes for patients (which also bring economic benefits of their own).

There is certainly no need to convene another ASCO panel, however, if the most positive conclusion is likely to be a call for randomized controlled trials (RCTs) before the Test can be endorsed. Such *pro forma* calls for clinical trials are tedious, at best, especially when those making the call have no intention of ever *funding* those RCTs.

It is ironic that often the very people calling most vociferously for RCTs have the greatest ability to perform such trials, i.e., scientists who reap the munificence of the large pharmaceutical companies.

In 2008, the American Cancer Society (ACS), for instance, had a cash and investment reserve of over one billion dollars,[432] yet to my knowledge not a single one of those dollars goes to chemosensitivity laboratories to improve their methods.

Time and again, FDA's requirement that new drugs actually be proven to extend overall survival has been waived in the case of cherished products of Big Pharma. (I have mentioned Avastin and breast cancer or Folotyn and peripheral T-cell lymphoma.)

But small laboratories, with very limited assets, are told that they need to produce multi-million dollar studies in order to gain acceptance.

In my opinion, advocates of the Test do not need to perform RCTs. They have every right to have their assays

treated according to long-established guidelines on clinical testing that have been in place for over half a century.
These are used to establish the accuracy and reliability of
laboratory assays, such as those for estrogen receptors
(ER) and prostate specific antigen (PSA).

Novel and onerous hurdles, such as providing proof
that use of the Test invariably leads to extended patient
survival, should not be put in the way of this, *and only
this*, form of testing. As I have said, this is a violation of
the bedrock principle of equal justice under the law.

In addition, Congress should strongly urge NCI to
allocate money specifically to revive its research program
in chemosensitivity assays The first item of business
should be systematically to compare the presently available Tests (including, of course, PCD-based tests) in terms
of their relative sensitivity, specificity, and positive and
negative predictive accuracies.

Some people may object that this would represent
political meddling in the scientific process. However, I
have found through my own experience as an advisor that
the National Institutes of Health (NIH) can be very
responsive to the wishes of the Congress.

The National Center for Complementary and Alternative Medicine (NCCAM) started as the Office of Alternative Medicine (OAM) in 1992 with a mere $2 million in
funding. It is no secret that NIH as a whole was initially
reluctant to take on the study of this controversial field.[433]

But by fiscal year (FY) 2010 the budget had grown sixty-fold, to $128.8 million.

It was mainly the intense interest of one Congressman, Sen. Tom Harkin (D-IA) that led to the present high level of support and interest. The same could happen with the Test.

Remember that the "scientific process," left to its own devices, has led to the current impasse, in which patented and expensive new drugs, procedures and tests are vigorously promoted by interested parties while older, less expensive but no less effective technologies are left in the dust.

Congress, through investigative hearings and specific funding suggestions, has the power to overcome this hugely expensive but socially destructive tendency to avoid chemosensitivity assays. It must act. When it does so, it should stipulate that the pioneers of the programmed cell death-based assays are included at every stage from the planning of studies to the disbursement of funds.

The Test has revolutionary potential. Its wide-scale use could transform oncology and put it for the first time on a truly customized basis. It is not necessary to wait for some putatively more accurate genomic test in order to implement the Test.

Regardless of the setbacks that have been encountered along the way, NCI should vigorously pursue this "Holy

Grail" of cancer diagnosis. *Indeed, short of a universal cure, one can hardly imagine a development that would be more beneficial to cancer patients than the wide-scale adoption of the Test.*

APPENDIX A

Labs Performing the Test

At the present time, almost all laboratories performing the Test require a living sample of tumor tissue. At most laboratories, this is about one gram of an individual's tumor, obtained fresh at the time of surgery or biopsy. Precision Therapeutics claims to need as little as two core needle biopsies (≥35 mg) or ascites or pleural fluid (≥100 cc). For some kinds of cancer, such as leukemia, most laboratories can work with a blood sample. Here is a list of some chemosensitivity laboratories in the US and abroad.

Anticancer, Inc.
7917 Ostrow St.
San Diego, CA 92111
Tel: 858-654-2555
Fax: 858-268-4175
E-mail: all@anticancer.com
Web: www.anticancer.com
Contact: Charlene Cooper, VP, COO
Li Tang, Business Development Manager
Director: R.M. Hoffman, MD

Cell Biolabs, Inc.
7758 Arjons Drive
San Diego, CA 92126
Tel: 858-271-6500
Toll-Free: 888-225-0505
Fax: 858-271-6514
General inquiries: info@cellbiolabs.com

DiaTech Oncology (Corporate Headquarters)
9208 Heritage Dr.
Brentwood, TN 37027
Tel: 877-434-2832 or 615-377-9668
Fax: 615-665-8730
Web: www.diatech-oncology.com
Email: info@diatech-oncology.com
Contact: R. Garry Latimer, President

DiaTech Oncology Clinical Laboratory
(Campus McGill University)
740 Dr. Penfield Ave Suite 4200
Montreal, QC Canada
H3A 1A4
Tel: 866-556-5356

Exiqon, Inc. (formerly Oncotech, Inc.)
15501 Red Hill Avenue
Tustin, CA 92780 USA
Tel: 800-576-6326 or 714-566-0420
Fax: 714-566-0421
Web: www.exiqon.com
Email: info@oncotech.com
Director: Doug Harrington
Some of their tests are done on pathology paraffin blocks.

Genomic Health, Inc. Corporate Headquarters
101 Galveston Drive
Redwood City, CA 94063
Tel: 650-556-9300
Fax: 650-556-1132 or 650-556-1073
Toll-free customer Service: 866-662-6897
Performs the Oncotype DX test

Genoptix Laboratory Facility
2110 Rutherford Rd.
Carlsbad, CA 92008
Tel: 760-268-6200 or 800-755-1605
Fax: 760-268-6201
Email General Inquiry: info@genoptix.com
Email Client Services: clientservices@genoptix.com
Fax Client Services: 888-755-1604
Director: Dr. Bashar Dabbas

Laboratory for Applied Neoplasia Research and
Cytostatics (L.A.N.C.E.)
Friedensplatz 16
D-53111 Bonn, Germany
Tel: +49-228-4335836
Fax: +49-228-4335837
Email: info@lance.de
Web: www.lance.de (English page available)
Tests available: ATP-TCA for many kinds of cancer
Contact: Christian Kurbacher, MD, PhD
Directors: Uwe Reinhold, MD, PhD, and
Ralf Reichelt, PhD.

Labor Dr. Limbach und Kollegen
Medizinisches Versorgungszentrum
Im Breitspiel 15 - 69126 Heidelberg
Germany
Tests: ATP luminesence and many other types
Works with practitioners, not directly with patients
Tel: +49-157-71628221
Fax: +49-6221-3432-110
Mobile: 0157 - 71628221
Web: www.labor-limbach.de (German only)
Director: Dr. Fritz Wosegien,
Schauinsland 24, 71642
Ludwigsburg, Germany
Tel: +49-71 41 5 12 12

Mosaic Laboratories, L.L.C.
12 Spectrum Pointe Drive
Lake Forest, CA 92630
Tel: 949-472-8000
Fax: 949-472-8855
Web: www.mosaiclabs.com
info@mosaiclabs.com
Contact: Chris Kirkwood

Precision Therapeutics, Inc.
2516 Jane Street
Pittsburgh, PA 15203
Tel: 514-398-5174 or 800-547-6165
Fax: 514-398-4939
Web sites: www.ptilabs.com
 www.chemofx.com
 www.precisiontherapeutics.com
Director: Jason Bush
Owner: Sean McDonald
Email: info@ptilabs.com or
info@precisiontherapeutics.com

Rational Therapeutics, Inc.
750 East 29th St.
Long Beach CA 90806
Tel: 562-989-6455
Fax: 562-989-8160
Web: www.rational-t.com
E-mail: Client.Services@RationalTherapeutics.com
Director: Robert A. Nagourney, MD

TherapySelect GmbH & Co. KG
Im Neuenheimer Feld 584
D-69120 Heidelberg
Germany
Tel.: +49-6221-8936-152
Fax: +49-6221-8936-153
Web: http://www.therapyselect.de/home.htm (German)
E-Mail: info@therapyselect.de
Tests: Biochip, Genchip
Chief scientific officer: Dr. Frank C. Kischkel, PhD
frank.kischkel@therapyselect.de

Weisenthal Cancer Group
16512 Burke Lane
Huntington Beach, CA 92649
Phone: 714-596-2100
Tel: 866-364-0011
Fax: 714-596-2110
Director: Larry Weisenthal, MD, PhD
Email: mail@weisenthal.org
Web: Weisenthalcancer.com and weisenthal.org (large atlas and other resources)

www.cancertest.org (blog for scientists and physicians concerning Individualized Tumor Response Testing (ITRT)
www.medpedia.com/users/110 (CV for Dr. Weisenthal)
Tests: Functional Tumor Cell Profiling (requires live tumor cells); EGFRx; DISC (Differential Staining Cytotoxicity); MTT Assay; ATP Assay; Resazurin Assay; Microvascular Viability (to determine drugs that will attack tumor vasculature, such as protein kinase inhibitors). Open Phase II Clinical Trial using FCP (Functional Cellomic Profiling)

APPENDIX B

Labs Analyzing CTCs

Biofocus Institute for Laboratory Medicine
Berghäuser Str. 295
45659 Recklinghausen, Germany
Tel.: +49 2361 3000-144 or +49-2361-3000-130
Fax: +49 2361 3000-162
Web: www.biofocus.de
Dr. med. Doris Bachg; Dr. med. Uwe Haselhorst;
Dr. Lothar Prix

Labor und Praxis Dr. med. Ulrich Pachmann
Kurpromenade 2
D-95448 Bayreuth, Germany
Tel: +49-921/850 200 (or -201) or +49 921 793 08 42
Fax: +49-921/850 203 or +49 921 78 77 94 55
Web: www.laborpachmann.de (only in German; they suggest using Google translator)
Owner/Director: Dr. med. Ulrich Pachmann
Technical Director: Dr. rer. nat. Ernst-Ludwig Stein
Contact: Henrike Freier
Email: tzb.freier_@_t-online.de
Test: MAINTRAC detects CTC, also chemosensitivity and resistance testing; developed by Prof. Katharina Pachmann

Research Genetic Cancer Centre (RGCC)

115 M. Alexandrou St.

53070 Filotas-Florina, Greece

Tel: +30-24630-42264

Fax: +30-24630-42265

Web: www.rgcc-genlab.com

Tests: Microarray sensitivity and resistance testing

REFERENCES

Note: Unwieldy URLs have been shortened and immortalized through the Website, www.tinyurl.com

---

[1] Von Hoff DD, Clark GM, Stogdill BJ, *et al.* Prospective clinical trial of a human tumor cloning system. *Cancer Res.* 1983;43:1926-1931.

[2] http://tinyurl.com/yzj4kxu

[3] Ibid.

[4] Elliott J. Almost a reality: prediction of drug effects on human cancers. *JAMA.* 1979;242:501-503, 508.

[5] Fruehauf JP and Bosquanet AG. *In vitro* determination of drug response: A discussion of clinical applications. In DeVita VJ, Jr., Hellman S, and Rosenberg, SA, eds. *PPO Updates to Cancer: Principles and Practice of Cancer Management*, vol. 7, Dec. 1993;7(12):1-13. Available at: http://tinyurl.com/39pssha

[6] Eissa, Saad and Shoman, Sohair. *Tumor Markers.* London: Chapman & Hall, 1998.

[7] Chu, Edward and DeVita, Vincent. Principles of Cancer Management: Chemotherapy. In: DeVita, VJ, Jr. Hellman, Samuel, Rosenberg, Steven A. (Eds.) *Cancer: Principles and Practice of Cancer Management,* 6th edition, Philadelphia: LWW, 2001, p. 302-306.

[8] http://tinyurl.com/ygxtl64

[9] Hwu P, Bedikian AY, Grimm EA. Challenges of chemosensitivity testing. *Clin Cancer Res.* 2006;12:5258-5259.

[10] Cree IA. Chemosensitivity and chemoresistance testing in ovarian cancer. Curr. Opin. *Obstet Gynecol.* 2009;21:39-43.

[11] http://www.cancer.gov/dictionary/?CdrID=45990

[12] http://tinyurl.com/23o5dnz

[13] Schrag D, Garewal HS, Burstein HJ, et al. American Society of Clinical Oncology Technology Assessment: Chemotherapy sensitivity and resistance assays. *J Clin Oncol.* 2004;22:3631-3638.

[14] Faguet, Guy. The War on Cancer: An Anatomy of Failure, A Blueprint for the Future. New York: Springer, 2006.

[15] Kolata, Gina. Lack of study volunteers hobbles cancer fight. *New York Times*, August 2, 2009.

[16] Tanjong-Ghogomu E, Tugwell P, Welch V. Evidence-based medicine and the Cochrane Collaboration. *Bull NYU Hosp Jt Dis.* 2009;67:198-205.

[17] www.virtualtrials.com

[18] http://www.htaj.com/faq.htm

[19] Hordijk-Trion M, Lenzen M, Wijns W, et al. Patients enrolled in coronary intervention trials are not representative of patients in clinical practice: results from the Euro Heart Survey on Coronary Revascularization. *Eur Heart J.* 2006;27:671-678.

[20] Shackley DC, Clarke NW. Impact of socioeconomic status on bladder cancer outcome. *Curr Opin Urol.* 2005;15:328-331.

[21] Sant M, Aareleid T, Berrino F, et al. EUROCARE-3: survival of cancer patients diagnosed 1990-94--results and commentary. *Ann Oncol.* 2003;14 Suppl 5:61-118.

[22] Antman K, Amato D, Wood W, et al. Selection bias in clinical trials. *J Clin Oncol.* 1985;3:1142-1147.

[23] Sharpe N. Clinical trials and the real world: selection bias and generalisability of trial results. *Cardiovasc Drugs Ther.* 2002;16:75-77.

[24] Herland K, Akselsen J, Skjønsberg OH, Bjermer L. How representative are clinical study patients with asthma or COPD for a larger "real life" population of patients with obstructive lung disease? *Respir Med.* 2005;99:11-19.

[25] Ramsey S, Scoggins J. Commentary: practicing on the tip of an information iceberg? Evidence of under-publication of registered clinical trials in oncology. *Oncologist.* 2008;13:925-929.

[26] Harris P, Takeda A, Loveman E, Hartwell D. Time to full publication of studies of anticancer drugs for breast cancer, and the potential for publication bias. *Int J Technol Assess Health Care.* 2010;26:110-116.

[27] Chu, Edward and DeVita, Vincent. Op. cit., p. 304.

[28] Chu, Edward and DeVita, Vincent. Op. cit., p. 302-306.

[29] http://tinyurl.com/y8cv2ls

[30] Latimer G, Presant CA, Hallquist A, Perree M, Agapitos D. The value of personalized treatment (Rx) planning (PTP): Cost savings (sav) by the microculture kinetic (MiCK) chemosensitivity (CS) assay, evidence from a large American self-insured company (ASIC). *J Clin Oncol.* 2009;27: Abstract e17541.

[31] Sikora K. Surrogate endpoints in cancer drug development. *Drug Discov Today.* 2002;7:951-956.

[32] Kaufmann SH. Paul Ehrlich: Founder of chemotherapy. *Nat Rev Drug Discov.* 2008;7:373.

[33] Canetti G, Froman S, Grosset J, *et al.* Mycobacteria: laboratory methods for testing drug sensitivity and resistance. *Bull World Health Organ.* 1963;29:565–578.

[34] Canetti G, Fox W, Khomenko A, *et al.* Advances in techniques of resting mycobacterial drug sensitivity, and the use of sensitivity tests in tuberculosis control programmes. *Bull World Health Organ.* 1969;41:21–43.

[35] Mendoza MT. What's new in antimicrobial susceptibility testing? *Phil J Microbiol Infect Dis.* 1998;27:113–115.

[36] Jones GB. From mustard gas to medicines: the history of modern cancer chemotherapy. *Chem Herit.* 1998;15:8-9, 40-42.

[37] Anonymous. Sensitivity tests for clinical cancer chemotherapy. *JAMA.* 1965;194:291.

[38] Knock F. Sensitivity tests for cancer chemotherapy. *Arch Surg.* 1965;91:376-385.

[39] Black MM, Opler SR, Speer FD. Observations on the reduction of triphenyl tetrazolium chloride by normal and malignant human tissue. *Am J Pathol.* 1950;26:1097-1102.

[40] Black MM, Speer FD. Further observations on the effects of cancer chemotherapeutic agents on the in vitro dehydrogenase activity of cancer tissue. *J Natl Cancer Inst.* 1954;14:1147-1158.

[41] Black MM, Speer FD. In vitro and clinical effects of urethane plus triethylene melamine on human breast cancer. *Surg Gynecol Obstet.* 1956;102:420-426.

[42] Ibid.

[43] Straus FH, Cheronis ND. Reducing enzyme systems in living mammalian tissue and neoplasms by triphenyl tetrazolium chloride. *Proc Inst Med Chic.* 1948;17:195.

[44] Black MM, Opler SR, Speer FD. Observations on the reduction of triphenyl tetrazolium chloride by normal and malignant human tissue. *Am J Pathol.* 1950;26:1097-1102.

[45] Carmichael J, DeGraff WG, Gazdar AF, Minna JD, Mitchell JB. Evaluation of a tetrazolium-based semiautomated colorimetric assay: assessment of chemosensitivity testing. *Cancer Res.* 1987;47:936-942.

[46] Ibid.

[47] Ibid.

[48] Alley MC, Scudiero DA, Monks A, *et al.* Feasibility of Drug Screening with Panels of Human Tumor Cell Lines Using a Microculture Tetrazolium Assay. *Cancer Res.* 1988;48:589-601.

[49] Mosmann T. Rapid colorimetric assay for cellular growth and survival: application to proliferation and cytotoxicity assays. *J Immunol Methods.* 1983;65:55-63.

[50] Denizot F, Lang R. Rapid colorimetric assay for cell growth and survival. Modifications to the tetrazolium dye procedure giving improved sensitivity and reliability. *J Immunol Methods.* 1986;89:271-277.

[51] Denizot F, Lang R. Op.cit.

[52] Sieuwerts AM, Klijn JG, Peters HA, Foekens JA. The MTT tetrazolium salt assay scrutinized: how to use this assay reliably to measure metabolic activity of cell cultures *in vitro* for the assessment of growth characteristics, IC50-values and cell survival. *Eur J Clin Chem Clin Biochem.* 1995;33:813-823.

[53] http://www.virtualtrials.com/assay.cfm

[54] Wright JL, Cobb JP, Gumport SL, *et al.* Investigation of the relation between clinical and tissue culture response to chemotherapeutic agents of human cancer. *N Engl J Med.* 1957;252:1207-1211.

[55] Dipaolo JA, Dowd JE. Evaluation of inhibition of human tumor tissue by cancer chemotherapeutic drugs with an in vitro test. *J Natl Cancer Inst.* 1961;27:807-815.

[56] Limburg H, Krabe M. Die Zuchtung von non schlichem Krebs gewebe in der Gewebekultun und seine Sensibilitatstestung gegen neuere Zytostatika.

Dtsch Sch Med Wochenschr. 1964;89:1938-1946.

[57] http://www.virtualtrials.com/assay.cfm

[58] Schrek R, Leithold SL, Friedman IA, Best WR. Clinical evaluation of an *in vitro* test for radiosensitivity of leukemic lymphocytes. *Blood.* 1962;20:432-442.

[59] Hinkley HJ, Bosanquet AG. The *in vitro* radiosensitivity of lymphocytes from chronic lymphocytic leukaemia using the differential staining cytotoxicity (DiSC) assay. I--Investigation of the method. *Int J Radiat Biol.* 1992;61:103-110.

[60] Hinkley HJ, Bosanquet AG. The *in vitro* radiosensitivity of lymphocytes from chronic lymphocytic leukaemia using the differential staining cytotoxicity (DiSC) assay. II--Results on 40 patients. *Int J Radiat Biol.* 1992;61:111-121.

[61] Schrek, R. Slide-chamber method to measure sensitivity of cells to toxic agents. *AMA Arch. Path.* 1958;66:569-576.

[62] McGuire, William P. Foreword to Köchli, OR, Seven, B-U, Haller, U. (Eds.) *Chemosensitivity Testing in Gynecologic Malignancies and Breast Cancer.* Basel: Karger, 1994.

[63] Poupon MF, Arvelo F, Goguel AF, *et al.* Response of small-cell lung cancer xenografts to chemotherapy: multidrug resistance and direct clinical correlates. *J. Natl. Cancer Inst.* 1993;85:2023-2029.

[64] http://tinyurl.com/ydl22gg

[65] Carney DN, Winkler CF. *In vitro* assays of chemotherapeutic sensitivity. *Important Adv Oncol.* 1985:78-103.

[66] Nagourney RA. Ex vivo programmed cell death and the prediction of response to chemotherapy. *Curr Treat Options Oncol.* 2006;7:103-110.

[67] Fruehauf JP and Bosquanet AG. Op cit.

[68] Gupta PB, Chaffer CL, Weinberg RA. Cancer stem cells: mirage or reality? *Nat Med.* 2009;15:1010-1012.

[69] Puck TT, Marcus PI. Action of x-rays on mammalian cells. *J Exp Med.* 1956;103:653-666.

[70] Salmon SE, Hamburger AW, Soehnlen B, *et al.* Quantitation of differential sensitivity of human-tumor stem cells to anticancer drugs. *N Engl J Med.* 1978;298:1321-1327.

[71] Fruehauf JP and Bosquanet AG. Op cit.

[72] http://www.virtualtrials.com/assay.cfm

[73] Link KH, Aigner KR, Kuehn W, Schwemmle K, Kern DH. Prospective correlative chemosensitivity testing in high-dose intraarterial chemotherapy for liver metastases. *Cancer Res.* 1986;46:4837-4840.

[74] Von Hoff DD, Casper J, Bradley E, *et al.* Association between human tumor colony-forming assay results and response of an individual patient's tumor to chemotherapy. *Am J Med.* 1981;70:1027-1041.

[75] Von Hoff DD, Clark GM, Stogdill BJ, *et al.* Prospective clinical trial of a human tumor cloning system. *Cancer Res.* 1983;43:1926-1931.

[76] Pavelic ZP, Slocum HK, Rustum YM, *et al.* Growth of cell colonies in soft agar from biopsies of different human solid tumors. *Cancer Res.* 1980;40:4151-4158.

[77] Sandbach J, Von Hoff DD, Clark G, Cruz AB, Obrien M. Direct cloning of human breast cancer in soft agar culture. *Cancer.* 1982;50:1315-1321.

[78] Schlag P, Wolfrum J, Vergani G, Schreml W, Herfarth C. [Growth of tumour-cell colonies from human solid tumours (author's transl)]. *Dtsch Med Wochenschr.* 1982;107:1173-1177.

[79] Dittrich C, Jakesz R, Wrba F, *et al.* The human tumour cloning assay in the management of breast cancer patients. *Br J Cancer.* 1985;52:197-203.

[80] Benard J, Da Silva J, Riou G. Culture of clonogenic cells from various human tumors: drug sensitivity assay. *Eur J Cancer Clin Oncol.* 1983;19:65-72.

[81] Touzet C, Ruse F, Chassagne J, *et al.* In vitro cloning of human breast tumour stem cells: influence of histological grade on the success of cultures. *Br J Cancer.* 1982;46:668-669.

[82] Elliott J. Op cit.

[83] Ibid.

[84] The Clinical Society. The retrogression of cancer. *The Hospital* (London). 1896;21:163.

[85] Baker M. Melanoma in mice casts doubt on scarcity of cancer stem cells. *Nature.* 2008;456:553.

[86] Kelly PN, Dakic A, Adams JM, Nutt SL, and Strasser A. Tumor growth need not be driven by rare cancer stem cells. *Science.* 2007;317, 337.

[87] Hoffman RM. *In vitro* sensitivity assays in cancer: a review, analysis, and prognosis. *J Clin Lab Anal.* 1991;5:133-143.

[88] Hirabayashi N, Nishiyama M, Yamaguchi M, *et al.* Effects of oxygen tension on tumor colony formations assessed by human tumor clonogenic assay. *Jpn J Surg.* 1986;16:148-151.

[89] Niyazi M, Niyazi I, Belka C. Counting colonies of clonogenic assays by using densitometric software. *Radiat Oncol.* 2007;2:4.

[90] Dahle J, Kakar M, Steen HB, Kaalhus O. Automated counting of mammalian cell colonies by means of a flat bed scanner and image processing. *Cytometry A.* 2004;60:182-188.

[91] Delgado JN, Gisvold O, Remers WA, eds. *Textbook of Organic, Medicinal and Pharmaceutical Chemistry.* Philadelphia: Lippincott, 1998.

[92] Aapro M. Op.cit.

[93] Carney DN, Winkler CF. *In vitro* assays of chemotherapeutic sensitivity. *Important Adv Oncol.* 1985:78-103.

[94] McGuire WP. Foreword to Köchli, OR, Seven, B-U, Haller, U., eds. *Chemosensitivity Testing in Gynecologic Malignancies and Breast Cancer.* Basel: Karger, 1994, p. vii.

[95] Aapro M. Clonogenic assays for gynecological malignancies. In: Köchli, OR, Seven, B-U, Haller, U., eds. *Chemosensitivity Testing in Gynecologic Malignancies and Breast Cancer.* Basel: Karger, 1994, pp. 24-29.

[96] McGuire, William P. Foreword to Köchli, OR, Seven, B-U, Haller, U., eds. *Chemosensitivity Testing in Gynecologic Malignancies and Breast Cancer.* Basel: Karger, 1994.

[97] Von Hoff DD, Clark GM, Stogdill BJ, *et al.* Prospective clinical trial of a human tumor cloning system. *Cancer Res.* 1983;43:1926-1931.

[98] Ibid.

[99] Hoffman RM. *In vitro* sensitivity assays in cancer: a review, analysis, and prognosis. *J Clin Lab Anal.* 1991;5:133-143.

[100] Hager, Tom. Cancer drug sensitivity test has problems. *JAMA.*1982; 248: 3079-3084.

[101] Ibid.

[102] Carney DN, Winkler CF. *In vitro* assays of chemotherapeutic sensitivity. *Important Adv Oncol.* 1985:78-103.

[103] Elliott J. Op cit.

[104] Selby P, Buick RN, Tannock I. A critical appraisal of the "human tumor stem-cell assay." *N Engl J Med.* 1983;308:129-134.

[105] Ibid.

[106] http://www.virtualtrials.com/assay.cfm

[107] http://www.virtualtrials.com/assay.cfm

[108] Selby, op. cit.

[109] Ajani JA, Blaauw AA, Spitzer G, *et al.* Differential cytotoxic activity of chemotherapy agents on colony-forming cells from human tumors and normal bone marrow *in vitro. Exp Hematol.* 1985;13 Suppl 16:95-100.

[110] Strauss E. Op.cit.

[111] Strauss E. Op.cit.

[112] Weisenthal, Larry. Personal communication, Dec. 17, 2009.

[113] http://www.virtualtrials.com/assay.cfm

[114] Von Hoff DD, Weisenthal L. *In vitro* methods to predict for patient response to chemotherapy. Adv Pharmacol Chemother. 1980;17:133-156.

[115] Weisenthal LM. Cell Culture Drug Resistance Testing (CCDRT), May 25, 2003. Available at: www.virtualtrials.com.

[116] Weisenthal LM, Lippman ME. Clonogenic and nonclonogenic *in vitro* chemosensitivity assays. *Cancer Treat Rep.* 1985;69:615-632.

[117] www.virtualtrials.com/assay.cfm

[118] http://www.thefreedictionary.com/Cancer

[119] http://tinyurl.com/ydb5quh

[120] http://tinyurl.com/3yuy69u

[121] Kerr JF, Wyllie AH, Currie AR. Apoptosis: a basic biological phenomenon with wide-ranging implications in tissue kinetics. *Br J Cancer.* 1972;26:239-257.

[122] Kerr JF. Shrinkage necrosis: a distinct mode of cellular death. *J Pathol.* 1971;105:13-20.

[123] Fletcher S. Genesis of apoptosis. *BMJ.* 1994;309:542-543.

[124] Clarke PG, Clarke S. Nineteenth century research on naturally occurring cell death and related phenomena. *Anat Embryol (Berl).* 1996;193:81-99.

[125] Beard J. On the early development of Lepidosteus osseus – preliminary notice. *Proc Roy Soc.* 1889;46:108-118.

[126] http://www.nih.gov/sigs/aig/Aboutapo.html

[127] Kerr JF, Wyllie AH, Currie AR. Op.cit.

[128] Reed JC. Dysregulation of apoptosis in cancer. *J Clin Oncol.* 1999;17:2941-2953.

[129] http://apoptosisinfo.com/

[130] http://tinyurl.com/ya8dm7k

[131] Golstein P. Cell death in us and others. *Science.* 1998;281:1283.

[132] Searle J, Lawson TA, Abbott PJ, Harmon B, Kerr JF. An electron-microscope study of the mode of cell death induced by cancer-chemotherapeutic agents in populations of proliferating normal and neoplastic cells. *J Pathol.* 1975;116:129-138.

[133] Reed JC. Dysregulation of apoptosis in cancer. *Cancer J Sci Am.* 1998;4 Suppl 1:S8-14.

[134] Nagourney RA. Ex vivo programmed cell death and the prediction of response to chemotherapy. *Curr Treat Options Oncol.* 2006;7:103-110.

[135] http://tinyurl.com/yagldyj

[136] Kamesaki S, Kamesaki H, Jorgensen TJ, *et al.* 1-bcl-2 protein inhibits etoposide-induced apoptosis through its effects on events subsequent to topoisomerase II-induced DNA strand breaks and their repair. *Cancer Res.* 1993;53:4251-4256.

[137] Fujiwara T, Grimm EA, Mukhopadhyay T, Cai DW, Owen-Schaub LB, Roth JA. A retroviral wild-type p53 expression vector penetrates human lung cancer spheroids and inhibits growth by inducing apoptosis. *Cancer Res.* 1993;53:4129-4133.

[138] Nagourney RA. Multidrug resistance in acute myeloid leukemia. *J Natl Cancer Inst.* 1991;83:1418-1419.

[139] Kravtsov VD, Fabian I. Automated monitoring of apoptosis in suspension cell cultures. *Lab Invest.* 1996;74:557-570.

[140] http://tinyurl.com/yhx7pj2

[141] http://tinyurl.com/yzsnbst

[142] Ibid.

[143] Ibid.

[144] http://tinyurl.com/yhx7pj2

[145] Lockshin RA, Williams CM. Programmed cell death—II. Endocrine potentiation of the breakdown of the intersegmental muscles of silkmoths. *J Insect Physiol.* 1964;10:643–649.

[146] Bursch W, Ellinger A, Gerner C, Fröhwein U, Schulte-Hermann R. Programmed cell death (PCD). Apoptosis, autophagic PCD, or others? *Ann N Y Acad Sci.* 2000;926:1-12.

[147] Frisch SM, Francis H. Disruption of epithelial cell-matrix interactions induces apoptosis. *J Cell Biol.* 1994;124:619-626.

[148] Bursch W, Ellinger A, Gerner C, Fröhwein U, Schulte-Hermann R. Op. cit.

[149] Nishizaki K, Anniko M, Orita Y, *et al.* Programmed cell death in the development of the mouse external auditory canal. *Anat Rec.* 1998;252:378-382.

[150] Lladó J, Calderó J, Ribera J, *et al.* Opposing effects of excitatory amino acids on chick embryo spinal cord motoneurons: excitotoxic degeneration or prevention of programmed cell death. *J Neurosci.* 1999;19:10803-10812.

[151] Fing SL and Cookson BT Apoptosis, pyroptosis, and necrosis: Mechanistic description of dead and dying eukaryotic cells. *Infect Immun.* 2005;73:1907-1916.

[152] Sperandio S, de Belle I, Bredesen DE. An alternative, non-apoptotic form of programmed cell death. *Proc Natl Acad Sci U.S.A.* 2000;97:14376-14381.

[153] Fink SL, Cookson BT. Apoptosis, pyroptosis, and necrosis: mechanistic description of dead and dying eukaryotic cells. *Infect Immun.* 2005;73:1907-1916.

[154] Abe Y, Yamamoto T, Sugiyama Y, *et al.* Apoptotic cells associated with Wallerian degeneration after experimental spinal cord injury: a possible mechanism of oligodendroglial death. *J Neurotrauma.* 1999;16:945-952.

[155] Dickler MN, Rugo HS, Eberle CA, *et al.* A phase II trial of erlotinib in combination with bevacizumab in patients with metastatic breast cancer. Clin. Cancer Res. 2008;14(23):7878-7883.

[156] Fruehauf JP and Bosquanet AG. *In vitro* determination of drug response: a discussion of clinical applications. In DeVita VJ, Jr., Hellman S, and Rosenberg, SA, eds. *PPO Updates to Cancer: Principles and Practice of Cancer Management*, vol. 7, Dec. 1993;7(12):1-13. Available at: www.caltri.org/pdf/FruehaufPPOUpd93.pdf

[157] Transcripts of the Medicare Coverage Advisory Committee (MCAC) Meeting, Baltimore, MD, November 15-16, 1999.

[158] Schrag D, Garewal HS, Burstein HJ, *et al.* Op cit.

[159] http://www.virtualtrials.com/assay.cfm

[160] http://www.virtualtrials.com/assay.cfm

[161] Von Hoff DD, Weisenthal L. *In vitro* methods to predict for patient response to chemotherapy. Adv Pharmacol Chemother. 1980;17:133-156.

[162] Fruehauf JP and Bosquanet AG. Op. cit.

[163] http://www.virtualtrials.com/assay.cfm

[164] Chu, Edward and DeVita, Vincent. Op. cit., p. 304.

[165] Weisenthal, personal communication, Dec. 17, 2009.

[166] http://www.virtualtrials.com/assay.cfm

[167] Von Hoff DD. He's not going to talk about *in vitro* predictive assays again, is he? *J. Natl. Cancer Inst.* 1990;82:96-101.

[168] Fruehauf JP and Bosquanet AG. Op. cit.

[169] Nagourney R. Chemosensitivity and resistance assays: A systematic review? *J Clin Oncol.* 2005;23:3640-3641.

[170] Fruehauf JP and Bosquanet AG. Op cit.

[171] Jensen EV, Block GE, Ferguson DJ, DeSombre ER. Estrogen receptors in breast cancer. *World J Surg.* 1977;1:341-342.

[172] Leung BS, Fletcher WS, Krippaehne WW. Estrogen receptor: a valid test for selection of breast cancer patients for endocrine ablation. *Surg Forum.* 1973;24:125-127.

[173] Andersen J, Bentzen SM, Poulsen HS. Relationship between radioligand binding assay, immunoenzyme assay and immunohistochemical assay for estrogen receptors in human breast

cancer and association with tumor differentiation. *Eur J Cancer Clin Oncol.* 1988;24:377-384.

[174] Pieslor PC, Gibson RE, Eckelman WC, *et al.* Three radioligands compared for determining cytoplasmic estrogen-receptor content of human breast carcinomas. *Clin. Chem.* 1982;28:532-537.

[175] Jensen EV, Block GE, Ferguson DJ, DeSombre ER. Estrogen receptors in breast cancer. World Journal of Surgery. 1977;1:341-342.

[176] Cikes M, Pettavel J. [Selection of patients with breast cancer with regard to endocrine therapy]. *Schweiz Med Wochenschr.* 1977;107:1645-1655.

[177] Edwards DP, Chamness GC, McGuire WL. Estrogen and progesterone receptor proteins in breast cancer. *Biochim. Biophys. Acta.* 1979;560:457-486.

[178] Chamness GC, Mercer WD, McGuire WL. Are histochemical methods for estrogen receptor valid? *J Histochem Cytochem.* 1980;28:792-798.

[179] http://www.cancertest.org/

[180] Yamashita H, Yando Y, Nishio M, *et al.* Immunohistochemical evaluation of hormone receptor status for predicting response to endocrine therapy in metastatic breast cancer. *Breast Cancer.* 2006;13:74-83.

[181] Yamashita. Op.cit.

[182] Southwest Oncology Group. http://tinyurl.com/yzm3btj

[183] Thompson IM, Pauler DK, Goodman PJ, *et al.* Prevalence of prostate cancer among men with a prostate-specific antigen level < or =4.0 ng per milliliter. *N Engl J Med.* 2004;350:2239-2246.

[184] Von Hoff DD. He's not going to talk about *in vitro* predictive assays again, is he? *J. Natl. Cancer Inst.* 1990;82:96-101.

[185] http://www.cancertest.org/?tag=colorectal-cancer

[186] http://tinyurl.com/y98gvv7

[187] http://www.bcrbiotech.com/

[188] Meitner PA. The fluorescent cytoprint assay: a new approach to in vitro chemosensitivity testing. *Oncology* (Williston Park, NY). 1991;5:75-81; discussion 81-82, 85, 88.

[189] Leone LA, Meitner PA, Myers TJ, *et al.* Predictive value of the fluorescent cytoprint assay (FCA): a retrospective correlation study of in vitro chemosensitivity and individual responses to chemotherapy. *Cancer Invest.* 1991;9:491-503.

[190] Rotman B, Teplitz C, Dickinson K, Cozzolino JP. Individual human tumors in short-term micro-organ cultures: chemosensitivity testing by fluorescent cytoprinting. *In Vitro Cell Dev Biol.* 1988;24:1137-1146.

[191] Abbas AK, Dorf ME, Karnovsky MJ, Unanue ER. The distribution of Ia antigens on the surfaces of lymphocytes. *J Immunol.* 1976;116:371-378.

[192] Nagourney RA, Kollin CA, Sommers B, Su Y-Z, Evans SS. Functional profiling of human tumors in primary culture: a platform for drug discovery & therapy selection. AACR abstract #1546, 2008.

[193] Ibid.

[194] Ibid.

[195] http://tinyurl.com/y8frm35

[196] Platoni, Kara. Thinking outside the cell. *East Bay Express.* 2007;30:10.

[197] Kern DH, Tanagawa N, Bertelson CA, *et al.* Heterogenicity of chemosensitivity response in human tumors. In: Salmon SE, Trent JM (Eds.). *Human Tumor Cloning.* Orlando: Grune and Stratton, 1984, p. 173.

[198] Nagourney, Robert. Personal communication, Jan. 7, 2010.

[199] Cristofanilli M, Mendelsohn J. Circulating tumor cells in breast cancer: Advanced tools for "tailored" therapy? *Proc Natl Acad Sci U.S.A.* 2006;103:17073-17074.

[200] Meng S, Tripathy D, Shete S, *et al.* HER-2 gene amplification can be acquired as breast cancer progresses. *Proc Natl Acad Sci U.S.A.* 2004;101:9393-9398.

[201] Kolata, Gina. Cancer fight: unclear tests for new drug. *New York Times*, April 19, 2010, page A1.

[202] Nagourney, Robert. Personal communication, Jan. 7, 2010.

[203] Ibid.

[204] Cortazar P, Gazdar AF, Woods E, *et al.* Survival of patients with limited-stage small cell lung cancer treated with individualized chemotherapy selected by *in vitro* drug sensitivity testing. *Clin Cancer Res.* 1997;3:741-747.

[205] Folkman J. Anti-angiogenesis: new concept for therapy of solid tumors. *Ann Surg.* 1972;175:409-416.

[206] American Cancer Society, Cancer Facts and Figures 2010.

[207] Greenberg PA, Hortobagyi GN, Smith TL, *et al.*: Long-term follow-up of patients with complete remission following combination chemotherapy for metastatic breast cancer. *J Clin Oncol.* 14:2197-205, 1996.

[208] Moss, RW. Cancer activism: gender, media and public policy. *New Scientist*, May 26, 2007. Available online: http://www.newscientist.com/

[209] Miller MC, Doyle GV, Terstappen LW. Significance of circulating tumor cells detected by the CellSearch system in patients with metastatic breast colorectal and prostate Cancer. *J Oncol.* 2010;2010:617421.

[210] De Lena M, De Palo GM, Bonadonna G, Beretta G, Bajetta E. [Therapy of metastatic mammary carcinoma with cyclophosphamide, methotrexate, vincristine and fluorouracil]. *Tumori.* 1973;59:11-24.

[211] Black MM and Speer FD. Further observations on the effects of cancer chemotherapeutic agents on the *in vitro* dehydrogenase activity of cancer tissue. *J Natl Cancer Inst.* 1954;14:1147-1158.

[212] Nagourney RA, Link JS, Blitzer JB, Forsthoff C, Evans SS. Gemcitabine plus cisplatin repeating doublet therapy in previously treated, relapsed breast cancer patients. *J. Clin. Oncol.* 2000;18:2245-2249.

[213] Whitworth, PW, Presant CA, Rutledge J, Hallquist A, Perree M, Agapitos D. Chemosensitivity (CS) of patient (pt) breast cancer (BrCa) cells *in vitro*: correlation with prior chemotherapy (CT) and implications for personalized treatment planning. *J Clin Oncol.* 2009;27, suppl; Abstract e11563.

[214] Whitworth, PW, Presant CA, Rutledge J, Hallquist A, Perree M, Agapitos D. Chemosensitivity (CS) of patient (pt) breast cancer (BrCa) cells *in vitro*: correlation with prior chemotherapy (CT) and implications for personalized treatment planning. *J Clin Oncol.* 2009;27, suppl; abstr e11563^.

[215] Kim H, Yom C, Moon B, *et al.* The use of an in vitro adenosine triphosphate-based chemotherapy response assay to predict chemotherapeutic response in breast cancer. *Breast.* 2008;17:19-26

[216] Ibid.

[217] American Cancer Society. *Cancer Facts and Figures—2010.*

[218] Dewey, Willis Alonzo. *Essentials of Homœopathic Materia Medica and Homœopathic Pharmacy.* 4th rev. ed., Philadelphia, Boericke & Tafel, 1908.

[219] Alderden RA, Hall MD, Hambley TW. The discovery and development of cisplatin. *J Chem Ed.* 2006;83:728-724.

[220] Nagourney RA, Brewer CA, Radecki S, *et al.* Phase II trial of gemcitabine plus cisplatin repeating doublet therapy in previously treated, relapsed ovarian cancer patients. *Gynecol. Oncol.* 2003;88:35-39.

[221] Ibid.

[222] Gallion H, Christopherson WA, Coleman RL, *et al.* Progression-free interval in ovarian cancer and predictive value of an ex vivo chemoresponse assay. Int. J. Gynecol. Cancer. 2006;16:194-201.

[223] Ibid.

[224] Cree IA, Kurbacher CM, Lamont A, Hindley AC, Love S. A prospective randomized controlled trial of tumour chemosensitivity assay directed chemotherapy versus physician's choice in patients with recurrent platinum-resistant ovarian cancer. *Anticancer Drugs.* 2007;18:1093-1101.

[225] http://tinyurl.com/ydgfyeh

[226] Ibid.

[227] Loizzi V, Chan JK, Osann K, *et al.* Survival outcomes in patients with recurrent ovarian cancer who were treated with chemoresistance assay-guided chemotherapy. *Am J Obstet Gynecol.* 2003;189:1301-1307.

[228] Cree IA, Kurbacher CM, Lamont A, Hindley AC, Love S. A prospective randomized controlled trial of tumour chemosensi-

tivity assay directed chemotherapy versus physician's choice in patients with recurrent platinum-resistant ovarian cancer. *Anticancer Drugs.* 2007;18:1093-1101.

[229] Salom EM, Penalver M, Homesley HD, *et al.* Can we increase response rate (RR) and overall survival (OS) by individualizing chemotherapy in ovarian cancer (OC): The role of a new chemotherapy (CT) induced apoptosis assay. *J Clin Oncol.* 2010;28:7s (suppl; abstr 5112).

[230] Ibid.

[231] Ballard KS, Homesley HD, Hodson C, *et al.* Endometrial carcinoma in vitro chemosensitivity testing of single and combination chemotherapy regimens using the novel microculture kinetic apoptosis assay: implications for endometrial cancer treatment. *J Gynecol Oncol.* 2010;21:45-49.

[232] Folkman J. Anti-angiogenesis: new concept for therapy of solid tumors. *Ann Surg.* 1972;175:409-416.

[233] http://tinyurl.com/y9tabal

[234] Ma WW, Adjei AA. Novel agents on the horizon for cancer therapy. *CA Cancer J Clin.* 2009;59:111-137.

[235] Keim, Brandon. FDA approves cancer drug that few can afford. i, Feb. 25, 2008 Accessed at: http://www.wired.com/

[236] Nagourney RA, Blitzer J, Deo E, *et al.* Functional profiling in stage IV NSCLC: A Phase II trial of individualized therapy. ASCO Abstract no. #e19079, June, 2009.

[237] Ramalingam SS, Maitland ML, Frankel P, *et al.* Carboplatin and Paclitaxel in combination with either vorinostat or placebo for first-line therapy of advanced non-small-cell lung cancer. *J Clin Oncol.* 2010;28:56-62.

[238] Hiramatsu A, Iwasaki Y, Koyama Y, *et al.* Phase II trial of weekly gemcitabine and split-dose cisplatin for advanced non-small-cell lung cancer. *Jpn J Clin Oncol.* 2009;39:779-783.

[239] Ihde DC. Small cell lung cancer. State-of-the-art therapy 1994. *Chest.* 1995;107(6 Suppl):243S-248S.

[240] Cortazar P, Gazdar AF, Woods E, *et al.* Survival of patients with limited-stage small cell lung cancer treated with individualized chemotherapy selected by *in vitro* drug sensitivity testing. *Clin Cancer Res.* 1997;3:741-747.

[241] Ibid.

[242] Slingluff CL, Chianese-Bullock KA, Bullock TN, *et al.* Immunity to melanoma antigens: from self-tolerance to immunotherapy. *Adv Immunol.* 2006;90:243-95.

[243] Weisenthal, Larry. Personal communication, March 2, 2010.

[244] Gimbel MI, Delman KA, Zager JS. Therapy for unresectable recurrent and in-transit extremity melanoma. *Cancer Control.* 2008;15:225-232.

[245] Legha SS. Durable complete responses in metastatic melanoma treated with interleukin-2 in combination with interferon alpha and chemotherapy. *Semin Oncol.* 1997;24(1 Suppl 4):S39-43.

[246] Pack & Livingston, *Treatment of Cancer and Allied Diseases*, NY 1940, p. 2501.

[247] Bosanquet AG, Johnson SA, Richards SM. Prognosis for fludarabine therapy of chronic lymphocytic leukaemia based on ex vivo drug response by DiSC assay. *Br J Haematol.* 1999;106:71-77.

[248] Ibid.

[249] Copur MS, Ledakis P, Muhvic J. Fludarabine for chronic lymphocytic leukemia. *N Engl J Med.* 2001;344:1166; author reply 1167-1168.

[250] http://tinyurl.com/yb7y22f

[251] Bosanquet AG, Johnson SA, Richards SM. Ibid.

[252] Ibid.

[253] Bosanquet, Andrew. Personal communication, December 27, 2009.

[254] http://tinyurl.com/yd744aw

[255] http://tinyurl.com/ykos64q

[256] Bosanquet AG. Correlations between therapeutic response of leukaemias and in-vitro drug-sensitivity assay. *Lancet.* 1991;337:711-714.

[257] Parkin DM, Bray F, Ferlay J, *et al.*: Estimating the world cancer burden: Globocan 2000. *Int J Cancer.* 2001;94:153-156.

[258] Cokgor I, Friedman HS, Friedman AH. Chemotherapy for adults with malignant glioma. *Cancer Invest.* 1999;17:264-272.

[259] Carmichael J, DeGraff WG, Gazdar AF, Minna JD, Mitchell JB. Evaluation of a tetrazolium-based semiautomated colorimetric assay: assessment of chemosensitivity testing. *Cancer Res.* 1987;47:936-942.

[260] Zhang JP, Shi HL, Sai K, *et al.* [Individualized chemotherapy based on drug sensitivity and resistance assay and MGMT protein expression for patients with malignant glioma--analysis of 42 cases] *Ai Zheng.* 2006;25:1533-1537.

[261] Pollack, Andrew. Questioning a $30,000-a-month cancer drug. *New York Times,* Dec. 4, 2009. Available online at: http://tinyurl.com/y9anyxm

[262] Latimer G, Presant CA, Hallquist Al, Perree M, Agapitos D. The value of personalized treatment (Rx) planning (PTP): Cost savings (sav) by the microculture kinetic (MiCK) chemosensitivity (CS) assay, evidence from a large American self-insured company (ASIC). *J Clin Oncol.* 2009;27:e17541.

[263] Ibid.

[264] Ibid.

[265] Schrag D, Garewal HS, Burstein HJ, *et al.* Op cit.

[266] http://www.virtualtrials.com/assay.cfm

[267] Samson DJ, Seidenfeld J, Ziegler K, Aronson N. Chemotherapy sensitivity and resistance assays: a systematic review. *J Clin Oncol.* 2004;22:3618-3630.

[268] http://jco.ascopubs.org/cgi/content/full/22/17/3631

[269] Schrag D, Garewal HS, Burstein HJ, *et al.* Op cit.

[270] Salmon SE, Hamburger AW, Soehnlen B, *et al.* Op cit.

[271] Von Hoff DD. He's not going to talk about *in vitro* predictive assays again, is he? *J Natl Cancer Inst.* 1990;82:96-101.

[272] http://www.usoncology.com/

[273] Von Hoff DD. Op cit.

[274] http://jco.ascopubs.org/cgi/content/full/23/15/3641

[275] Fruehauf JP, Alberts DS. In vitro drug resistance versus chemosensitivity: two sides of different coins. *J Clin Oncol.* 2005;23:3641-3643; author reply 3646-3648.

[276] Nagourney R. Chemosensitivity and resistance assays: A systematic review? *J Clin Oncol.* 2005;23:3640-3641.

[277] Cortazar P, Johnson BE. Review of the efficacy of individualized chemotherapy selected by *in vitro* drug sensitivity testing for patients with cancer. *J Clin Oncol.* 1999;17:1625.

[278] John P. Fruehauf. *In vitro* drug resistance versus chemosensitivity: Two sides of different coins. *J Clin Oncol.* 2005;23:3641-3643.

[279] Kent-Smith BT. Overuse of popular words in scientific communications: the robust apoptosis paradigm shift. *Clin Experiment Ophthalmol.* 2007;35:499.

[280] Scharg, op.cit.

[281] Nagourney R. Chemosensitivity and resistance sssays: A systematic review? *J Clin Oncol.* 2005;23:3640-3641.

[282] Ibid.

[283] Ibid.

[284] Ibid.

[285] Kim H, Yom C, Moon B, *et al.* The use of an in vitro adenosine triphosphate-based chemotherapy response assay to predict chemotherapeutic response in breast cancer. *Breast.* 2008;17:19-26.

[286] Angioli, Roberto, et al. (Eds.). Chemotherapy for Gynecological Neoplasms: Current Therapy and Novel Approaches. New York: Marcel Dekker, 2004, p. 50.

[287] Nagourney R. Op. cit.

[288] http://tinyurl.com/yz9t8su

[289] http://www.vicc.org/news/?p=504

[290] http://tinyurl.com/y8w8qn7

[291] http://tinyurl.com/y9aaox5

[292] Fruehauf JP, Alberts DS. Op. cit.

[293] Nagourney R. Op. cit.

[294] Wieand HS. Chemotherapy sensitivity and response assays: Are the ASCO guidelines for clinical trial design too restrictive? *J Clin Oncol.* 2005;23:3643-3644; author reply 3646-3648.

[295] Nagourney RA, Link J, Blitzer J, *et al.*: Gemcitabine plus cisplatin repeating doublet therapy in previously treated, relapsed breast cancer patients. *J Clin Oncol.* 2000;18:2245-2249.

[296] Ibid.

[297] http://tinyurl.com/282tjrp

[298] http://tinyurl.com/yg84nof

[299] http://tinyurl.com/y8j6e28

[300] Samson DJ, Seidenfeld J, Ziegler K, Aronson N. Op. cit.

[301] Lu JJ, Brady LW. (eds.) *Radiation Oncology: An Evidence-Based Approach.* Berlin: Springer, 2008.

[302] Op.cit., p. 213.

[303] Op.cit., p. 303.

[304] Miller K, Wang M, Gralow J, *et al.* Paclitaxel plus bevacizumab versus paclitaxel alone for metastatic breast cancer. *N Engl J Med.* 2007;357:2666-2676.

[305] Miller KD, Chap LI, Holmes FA, *et al.* Randomized phase III trial of capecitabine compared with bevacizumab plus capecitabine in patients with previously treated metastatic breast cancer. *J Clin Oncol.* 2005;23:792-799.

[306] Baar J, Silverman P, Lyons J, *et al.* A vasculature-targeting regimen of preoperative docetaxel with or without bevacizumab for locally advanced breast cancer: impact on angiogenic biomarkers. *Clin Cancer Res.* 2009;15:3583-3590.

[307] http://tinyurl.com/yduqwlw

[308] Pollack, Andrew. FDA panel urges limits for Avastin. *New York Times,* July 20, 2010.

[309] http://www.gene.com/gene/features/asco/

[310] http://tinyurl.com/26zts4

[311] Weisenthal, *Letter to Jeter, op.cit.*

[312] Thucydides, *History of the Peloponnesian War,* translated into English by Benjamin Jowett, 2nd ed., Oxford: Clarendon Press, 1900.

[313] http://tinyurl.com/y89zf4q

[314] Anonymous. *Clinical Operations: Accelerating Trials, Allocating Resources and Measuring Performance,* Cutting Edge Information, 2006. Accessed at: http://www.cuttingedgeinfo.com/clinical-trials/

[315] National Cancer Institute. NCI Budget Snapshot, Accessed at: www.cancer.gov/aboutnci/servingpeople/snapshot

[316] Weisenthal, Larry. Frequently-asked questions relating to cell culture drug resistance testing (CCDRT). Accessed at http://www.weisenthal.org/faqw.htm

[317] Moss, RW. *The Cancer Industry.* Lemont, PA: Equinox Press, 2000.

[318] Brown E, Markman M: Tumor chemosensitivity and chemoresistance assays. *Cancer.*1996;77:1020-1025.

[319] Fruehof J. *In vitro* drug resistance versus chemosensitivity: Two sides of different coins. *J Clin Oncol.* 2005;23:3641-3643.

[320] http://www.virtualtrials.com/assay.cfm

[321] http://www.virtualtrials.com/assay.cfm

[322] Girion, Lisa. Blue Cross praised employees who dropped sick policyholders, lawmaker says. *Los Angeles Times*, June 17, 2009.

[323] Ibid.

[324] Ibid.

[325] Faguet, Guy. Op cit.

[326] Leaf, Clifford. Why we're losing the war on cancer. *Fortune.* 2004;149:76-97.

[327] Moss, Ralph W. *Questioning Chemotherapy.* Lemont, PA: Equinox Press, 1996.

[328] American Cancer Society. *Cancer Facts and Figures—2010.* Accessed at www.cancer.org

[329] http://tinyurl.com/yfmbo6d

[330] Reck M, von Pawel J, Zatloukal P, *et al.* Phase III trial of cisplatin plus gemcitabine with either placebo or bevacizumab as first-line therapy for nonsquamous non-small-cell lung cancer: AVAiL. *J Clin Oncol.* 2009;27:1227-1234.

[331] Ibid.

[332] Sandler A, Gray R, Perry MC, *et al.* Paclitaxel-carboplatin alone or with bevacizumab for non-small-cell lung cancer. *N Engl J Med.* 2006;355: 2542-2550.

[333] Ibid.

[334] Ibid.

[335] Anonymous. Stage IV non-small cell lung cancer. National Cancer Institute Web site. Accessed at http://tinyurl.com/yfmbo6d

[336] Fruehauf JP and Bosquanet AG. Op. cit.

[337] Goozner, Merrill. Cure cancer? Not without a course correction. *Gooz News*, June 29, 2009. Accessed at: http://www.gooznews.com/node/2981

[338] Ibid.

[339] Ibid.

[340] Williams, Roger J. *Biochemical Individuality*. New York: McGraw Hill, 1998.

[341] Le Lorier J, Grégoire G. Meta-analysis and the meta-epidemiology of clinical research. Comments on paper by author of editorial were unwarranted. BMJ. 1998;316:311-312.

[342] Ibid.

[343] Takita H, Marabella PC, Edgerton F, Rizzo D. cis-Dichlorodiammineplatinum(II), adriamycin, cyclophosphamide, CCNU, and vincristine in non-small cell lung carcinoma: a preliminary report. *Cancer Treat Rep.* 1979;63:29-33.

[344] http://tinyurl.com/yzwuo3b

[345] Anonymous. Pipeline Insight: Molecular Targeted Cancer Therapies - More Pipeline Activity, Less Product Differentiation, Datamonitor, Nov., 2008

[346] Strauss, Evelyn. *Op.cit.*

[347] Taylor, Nick. Record R&D investment in US. *Decision News Media SAS*, March 27, 2008.

[348] Anonymous. Clinical Trial Recruitment Strategies: Optimizing Patient Recruitment and Retention in Late Stage Clinical Trials. Business Insights. Jan. 1, 2010. Available at: www.marketresearch.com

[349] Barnes, Kirsty. New Research offers CRO market snapshot. *Outsourcing-Pharma,* November 22, 2007.

[350] Anonymous. Riding the wave. *Pharmaceutical Executive Europe, FOCUS Oncology,* September 2007, pp. 3-5.

[351] http://www.quintiles.com/

[352] http://www.quintiles.com/therapeutic-areas/oncology/

[353] http://tinyurl.com/yamgpd7

[354] Wieand HS. Op. cit.

[355] Murthy VH, Krumholz HM, Gross CP. Participation in cancer clinical trials: race-, sex-, and age-based disparities. *JAMA.* 2004;291:2720-2726.

[356] Tournoux C, Katsahian S, Chevret S, Levy V. Factors influencing inclusion of patients with malignancies in clinical trials. *Cancer.* 2006;106:258-270.

[357] Grunfeld E, Zitzelsberger L, Coristine M, Aspelund F. Barriers and facilitators to enrollment in cancer clinical trials: qualitative study of the perspectives of clinical research associates. *Cancer.* 2002;95:1577-1583.

[358] Castel P, Négrier S, Boissel J. Why don't cancer patients enter clinical trials? A review. *Eur J Cancer.* 2006;42:1744-1748.

[359] Cox K, McGarry J. Why patients don't take part in cancer clinical trials: an overview of the literature. *Eur J Cancer Care (Engl).* 2003;12:114-122.

[360] Hussain-Gambles M, Leese B, Atkin K, *et al.* Involving South Asian patients in clinical trials. *Health Technol Assess.* 2004;8:1-109.

[361] Lara PN, Higdon R, Lim N, *et al.* Prospective evaluation of cancer clinical trial accrual patterns: identifying potential barriers to enrollment. *J Clin Oncol.* 2001;19:1728-1733.

[362] Campbell MK, Snowdon C, Francis D, *et al.* Recruitment to randomised trials: strategies for trial enrollment and participation study. The STEPS study. *Health Technol Assess.* 2007;11:iii, ix-105.

[363] DeAngelis CD, Drazen JM, Frizelle FA, *et al.* Clinical trial registration: a statement from the International Committee of Medical Journal Editors. *Arch Otolaryngol Head Neck Surg.* 2005;131:479-480.

[364] http://tinyurl.com/yaq46zg

[365] Anonymous. Chemotherapy kickbacks influence prescribing patterns. *Cancer Monthly.* Dec. 10, 2007. Accessed at: http://tinyurl.com/22c85g

[366] http://tinyurl.com/yaq46zg

[367] Ibid.

[368] Jacobson M, O'Malley AJ, Earle CC, *et al.* Does reimbursement influence chemotherapy treatment for cancer patients? *Health Aff (Millwood).* 2006;25:437-443.

[369] Jacobson M, O'Malley AJ, Earle CC, *et al.* Does Reimbursement Influence Chemotherapy Treatment For Cancer Patients? *Health Aff.* 2006;25:437-443.

[370] http://patternsofcare.com/2005/1/editor.htm

[371] http://tinyurl.com/yc7aj8o

[372] www.adjuvantonline.com

[373] http://tinyurl.com/y887ubg

[374] U.S. Department of Health and Human Services. Excessive medicare payment for prescription drugs, Pub. No. OEI-03-97-00290. Washington: U.S. Government Printing Office, Dec. 1997.

[375] DHHS, Medicare reimbursement of prescription drugs. Pub. No. OEI-03-00-00310. Washington: GPO, December 2001.

[376] U.S. Government Accountability Office. Medicare: payments for covered outpatient drugs exceed provider's cost, Pub. No. GAO-01-1118. Washington: GPO, September 2001.

[377] http://tinyurl.com/yzzgy3o

[378] http://tinyurl.com/yzdjsnb

[379] Peck, Peggy. ASCO leadership pulls out all stops in campaign for Quality Cancer Care Preservation Act. *Oncology Times*. 2003;25:7-8. Accessed from: http://tinyurl.com/yz7dwvj

[380] Jacobson M, Earle CC, Price M, Newhouse JP. How Medicare's payment cuts for cancer chemotherapy drugs changed patterns of treatment. *Health Aff*. 2010:hlthaff.2009.0563.

[381] Abelson, Reed. Doctors recouped cuts in Medicare pay, study finds. *New York Times*, June 16, 2010.

[382] Ibid.

[383] http://tinyurl.com/y8nkqfk

[384] Berenson, Alex. Incentives limit any savings in treating cancer. *New York Times*, June 12, 2007.

[385] Ibid.

[386] Pachmann, Katharina. The Maintrac analysis of circulating tumor cells allows direct monitoring of the effect of adjuvant chemotherapy in breast cancer patients. *Proc Am Soc Clin Oncol*. 2001;20: Abstract 1786.

[387] Gasent Blesa JM, Alberola Candel V, Esteban González E, *et al*. Circulating tumor cells in breast cancer: methodology and clinical repercussions. *Clin Transl Oncol*. 2008;10:399-406.

388 Camara O, Rengsberger M, Egbe A, *et al.* The relevance of circulating epithelial tumor cells (CETC) for therapy monitoring during neoadjuvant (primary systemic) chemotherapy in breast cancer. *Ann. Oncol.* 2007;18:1484-1492.

389 Lobodasch K, Fröhlich F, Rengsberger M, *et al.* Quantification of circulating tumour cells for the monitoring of adjuvant therapy in breast cancer: an increase in cell number at completion of therapy is a predictor of early relapse. *Breast.* 2007;16:211-218.

390 Pachmann K, Clement JH, Schneider C, *et al.* Standardized quantification of circulating peripheral tumor cells from lung and breast cancer. *Clin. Chem. Lab. Med.* 2005;43:617-627.

391 Pachmann K, Dengler R, Lobodasch K, *et al.* An increase in cell number at completion of therapy may develop as an indicator of early relapse: quantification of circulating epithelial tumor cells (CETC) for monitoring of adjuvant therapy in breast cancer. *J Cancer Res Clin Oncol.* 2008;134:59-65.

392 Meng S, Tripathy D, Frenkel EP, *et al.* Circulating tumor cells in patients with breast cancer dormancy. Clin. Cancer Res. 2004;10:8152-8162.

393 Carlson, Robert H. AACR Annual Meeting:

finding and identifying disseminated tumor cells as biomarkers for solid cancers. *Oncology Times,* 2005;27:10-11.

394 Morgan TM, Lange PH, Porter MP, *et al.* Disseminated tumor cells in prostate cancer patients after radical prostatectomy and without evidence of disease predicts biochemical recurrence. Clin. Cancer Res. 2009;15:677-683.

395 National Cancer Institute. Putting circulating tumor cells to the test. *Cancer Bulletin.* 2009 (Dec. 15);6:24. Accessed at: http://tinyurl.com/ydjpfzm

[396] National Cancer Institute. Putting circulating tumor cells to the test. *Cancer Bulletin.* 2009;6:24. Accessed at: http://tinyurl.com/ydjpfzm

[397] Camara O, Kavallaris A, Nöschel H, *et al.* Seeding of epithelial cells into circulation during surgery for breast cancer: the fate of malignant and benign mobilized cells. *World J Surg Oncol.* 2006;4:67.

[398] Ibid.

[399] Ibid.

[400] Pachmann K. Personal communication, June 6, 2010.

[401] Pachmann K, Stein E-L, Spitz G, Schill E, Pachmann U. Chemosensitivity testing of circulating epithelial Cells (CETC) in breast cancer patients and correlation to clinical outcome. *Cancer Res.* 2009; 69(Suppl):606s, SABCS poster #2044.

[402] Giesing M, Schütz A, Prix L, *et al.* Molecular staging of solid cancer and of minimal residual tumour cells: A novel approach to cancer patient management. [No publication venue or date given.]

[403] (Personal communication, Feb. 3, 2010).

[404] Pachmann U, Pachmann K. Method for determining the concentration of vital epithelial tumor cells in a bodily fluid. United State Patent No. US 7,615,358 B2, Nov. 10, 2009, section 1.

[405] Müller V, Alix-Panabières C, Pantel K. Insights into minimal residual disease in cancer patients: Implications for anti-cancer therapies. *Eur J Cancer.* 2010;46:1189-1197.

[406] Lőrincz T, Tóth J, Badalian G, Tímár J, Szendrői M. HER-2/neu genotype of breast cancer may change in bone metastasis. *Pathol Oncol Res.* 2006;12:149-152.

[407] Meng S, Tripathy D, Frenkel EP, *et al.* Circulating tumor cells in patients with breast cancer dormancy. *Clin Cancer Res.* 2004;10(24):8152-8162.

[408] Cristofanilli M, Mendelsohn J. Circulating tumor cells in breast cancer: Advanced tools for "tailored" therapy? *Proc Natl Acad Sci U.S.A.* 2006;103:17073-17074.

[409] Ibid.

[410] http://www.virtualtrials.com/assay.cfm

[411] http://tinyurl.com/ybfacr5

[412] American Society for Clinical Oncology (ASCO) Press Release. Personalized cancer medicine: Advances in cancer vaccines and targeted therapies. May 31, 2009.

[413] http://www.ced.osu.edu/PersonalizedHealthCare/

[414] Collins, Francis S. The Language of Life: DNA and the Revolution in Personalized Medicine. New York: Harper, 2010.

[415] Niederhuber, John. The dawn of personalized oncology. *Cancer Bulletin*, August 19, 2008. Accessed at: http://www.cancer.gov/

[416] Sparber A, Bauer L, Curt G, *et al.* Use of complementary medicine by adult patients participating in cancer clinical trials. *Oncol Nurs Forum.* 2000;27:623-630.

[417] Ibid.

[418] http://www.cancertest.org/?tag=colorectal-cancer

[419] Puck TT, Marcus PI. 1Action of x-rays on mammalian cells. *J Exp Med.* 1956;103:653-666.

[420] Schrek R, Best WR, Stefani S. Relationship between in vitro and in vivo radiosensitivity of lymphocytes in chronic lymphocytic leukemia. *Acta Haematol.* 1988;80:129-133.

[421] Hinkley HJ, Bosanquet AG. The in vitro radiosensitivity of lymphocytes from chronic lymphocytic leukaemia using the differential staining cytotoxicity (DiSC) assay. I--Investigation of the method. *Int J Radiat Biol.* 1992;61:103-110.

[422] Hinkley HJ, Bosanquet AG. The in vitro radiosensitivity of lymphocytes from chronic lymphocytic leukaemia using the differential staining cytotoxicity (DiSC) assay. II—Results on 40 patients. *Int J Radiat Biol.* 1992;61:111-121.

[423] Comby E, Andre I, Troussard X, *et al.* In vitro evaluation of B-CLL cells apoptotic responses to irradiation. *Leuk Lymphoma.* 1999;34:159-166.

[424] Aapro, MS. Op.cit., p 24.

[425] Schrag D, Garewal HS, Burstein HJ, *et al.* Op cit.

[426] http://tinyurl.com/ycc8f2v

[427] http://tinyurl.com/yewvukh

[428] Thompson CA. FDA approves pralatrexate for treatment of rare lymphoma. *Am J Health Syst Pharm.* 2009;66:1890.

[429] Pollack, Andrew. Questioning a cancer drug that costs $30,000 a month. *New York Times*, Dec. 4, 2009.

[430] Ibid.

[431] Pollack, Andrew. F.D.A. approves 'vaccine' to fight prostate cancer, *New York Times*, April 29, 2010, page A13.

[432] http://tinyurl.com/ygkrdxs

[433] Angier, Natalie. U.S. opens the door just a crack to alternative forms of medicine. *New York Times.* January 10, 1993, page A22.

INDEX